To "Uncle Larry" Lundgren —
my first and best mentor —
thanks for everything!

Del Scott

Engineering Foundation Conferences

FRONTIERS

IN

INDUSTRIAL PROCESS TOMOGRAPHY

Proceedings of the the Engineering Foundation Conference held at The Cliffs
Shell Beach, California
October 29 - November 1995

Edited by

David M. Scott
Du Pont Company

Richard A. Williams
University of Exeter

Published by

Engineering Foundation
345 East 47th Street
New York, NY 10017

Table of Contents

Preface

Industrial processes are often controlled using "simple" process measurements (such as temperature, pressure, flow rate, or level) at one or more points in the process flowsheet. The amount of information contained in such measurements is minimal, and in some cases (such as multiphase flow) there are no adequate sensors. In order to develop a better understanding of certain chemical processes, a more sophisticated approach is needed. Such an approach is provided by the interdisciplinary field of process tomography, which combines recent developments in sensor technology with tomographic reconstruction techniques.

Tomographic imaging provides hitherto inaccessible data allowing dynamic behavior to be measured, modeled and controlled. Process tomography can increase the efficiency of industrial systems through improved equipment design, process control, development of fluid-flow and process models, multi-phase flow monitoring, and quality assurance of manufactured products. Environmental monitoring of groundwater movement, airborne dispersions and soil remediation applications are also enabled by this new technology.

Over the last five years there has been a rapid growth in this field. For example, in the European Union the strategic importance of the technology has been recognized by funding a major process engineering initiative to form integrated research networks of over 300 academic and industrial researchers. This group continues to expand. In the United Kingdom the Engineering and Physical Sciences Research Council (EPSCR, formerly SERC) has also targeted the area for priority funding for development of multiphase flow and separation modelling. In the USA significant expertise exists in the areas of Computed Tomography, impedance tomography, reconstruction and image analysis.

In order to foster world-wide communication between workers in this rapidly-developing area, the Engineering Foundation agreed to sponsor an international conference from October 29 to November 3, 1995 in San Luis Obispo, California. We believe that this conference, "Frontiers in Industrial Process Tomography", is the first truly international meeting devoted exclusively to this topic (the recent ECAPT meetings, for example, were primarily limited to participants from EC countries). In preparation for this significant event, we have prepared the present volume.

Although this book will serve as the conference proceedings, it is not simply a compilation of preprints of all the conference papers. Instead, we have attempted to assemble a concise text that surveys the state of the art from its technology to its applications. Most of the chapters in this volume are based on one or more abstracts that were submitted to the conference. The keynote addresses are included, and other manuscripts were solicited on the basis of either the breadth of coverage (as in the background chapters on technology) or the industrial relevance of the application. The final choice was based on which topics could be combined to make a coherent text. Due to space and time constraints, we had to limit the number of chapters; however, the appendix includes all of the abstracts received to date for the lectures and discussion papers (posters) that will be presented at the conference.

As in any multiply-authored text, there is bound to be some repetition of material, particularly in over-lapping subject areas. We have made every effort to hold such repetition to a minimum. The manuscripts were reviewed by other contributors to the volume and also by the conference Organizing Committee. In the editing phase, we have tried to impose as much uniformity as possible. We feel that the resulting volume is of better quality than one normally finds in pre-conference proceedings. It is our hope that the readers will agree.

A number of individuals have had a share in the preparing of this text, and we would like to recognize their efforts. The conference Organizing Committee helped us to decide which topics to include, and many of them also provided chapter contributions. Members were Prof. J. Ch. Bolomey, Dr. W. Daily, Dr. F. J. Dickin,

Dr. T. Dyakowski, Mr. R. B. Edwards, Prof. R. G. Green, Dr. J. S. Halow, Dr. J. Hooper, Dr. B. S. Hoyle, Prof. D. Isaacson, Dr. H. K. Kytömaa, Prof. F. Mesch, Prof. J. D. Miller, and Dr. E. J. Morton. Ms. Maggie Clark kept track of the abstracts and provided a vital communication link between the editors. In addition, we thank the contributors to this volume not only for taking the time to record their observations and views, but also for delivering their typescripts in time for us to meet an ambitious publication schedule.

Finally, we would like to acknowledge the assistance and sponsorship of the Engineering Foundation and the American Institute of Chemical Engineers. Additional sponsors were the Engineering and Physical Sciences Research Council (U.K.), the National Science Foundation, Unilever Research, the Institute of Chemical Engineers, and the Particle Technology Subject Group (I. Chem. E.).

June, 1995

David M. Scott   Richard A. Williams
Wilmington, Delaware, USA   Redruth, Cornwall, U.K.

Chapter 1

Introduction to Process Tomography

David M. Scott
Du Pont Central Research and Development
E. I. du Pont de Nemours and Co. (Inc.)
Experimental Station, E357
Wilmington, Delaware 19880-0357 USA

1. Beginnings

Tomography is an interdisciplinary field concerned with obtaining cross-sectional, two-dimensional images of three-dimensional objects. Its beginnings date back to 1917, when Radon [1] demonstrated that any N-dimensional object can be "reconstructed" from an infinite number of (N-1)-dimensional "projections". Such projections are analogous to ordinary radiographs, which "collapse" a 3-D object onto a 2-D image. By combining a large number of these radiographs, it is possible to determine the 3-D internal structure of the object.

The widespread use of tomography as a practical tool did not happen until after the development of the EMI Head Scanner in the 1960's [2]. This device used a computer to reconstruct the image from projection data, a technique now known as Computed Tomography (CT). The most prevalent use of tomography is still in medical applications, and much of the modern tomographic technology is derived from medical systems (Electrical Impedance Tomography [3] is one example). However, since the early 1980's there has been a growing acceptance of tomographic imaging in a number of diverse fields. Industrial nondestructive evaluation (NDE) applications of tomography include the examination of structural ceramics, castings, and small jet engines [4]. Tomographic reconstruction techniques have been used to visualize the structure of plasma in tokamak experiments [5], and tomography based on capacitive or impedance sensing has been used to study fluidization in gas-fluidized beds [6] and two-component flow through pipes [7]. Typical application areas of tomography are shown in Table 1.

Computed Tomography :	NDE, Medical applications
Process Tomography :	Chemical Engineering applications
Impedance Tomography :	Biomedical applications
Seismic Tomography :	Geophysics
Acoustic Tomography :	Oceanography
Synthetic Aperture Radar :	Astronomy, Astrophysics

Table 1 Typical application areas of tomography

The present volume examines the technology and industrial applications of process tomography, which includes some aspects of the other tomography areas. In this context, "process tomography" refers to any tomographic method used to measure the internal state of a chemical process (e.g., material distribution in a reactor, multiphase flow fields in piping, or concentration uniformity in mixers). Process tomography techniques include computed tomography, electrical methods (impedance, capacitance, and inductance tomography), positron emission tomography (PET), optical tomography, microwave tomography, acoustic methods, and many other modalities.

Industry is interested in process tomography primarily because improved understanding and control of a chemical process requires information about the physical state of the material involved. Process tomography provides an entirely new "window" for observing chemical processes, often in real-time, at a lower system cost than many common commercial analyzers. Tomographic techniques can measure quantities such as the flow rate or solids concentration of material flowing through a pipeline and the distribution of material inside a chemical reactor or a mixer. This type of information is not usually obtainable with the sensors traditionally used by the chemical engineer, particularly in the case of multiphase flows. Therefore these techniques promise a better understanding of the flow of material through the plant, and the data can be used to design better process equipment and to control certain processes to maximize yield and quality. Additional applications of process tomography will be listed below.

2.   Technology

Although tomographic techniques vary widely in their instrumentation and applications, all of them are characterized by a common two-step approach to the imaging process: first they gather projection data based on some physical sensing mechanism, then they reconstruct a cross sectional image from the projections. The term "projection" has a specific meaning in tomography; for the moment, a projection can be visualized as type of radiograph of the process vessel. The related concept of reconstruction will be discussed in more detail in Chapter 9.

It is an axiom of tomography that many projections are needed to reconstruct the interior volume or cross-section of an object. This requirement can be illustrated with an example taken from x-ray Computed Tomography, wherein a parallel-beam projection is made of a pipe containing a two-component mixture. A collimated beam of radiation from the source is attenuated as it passes through the pipe walls and the mixture. The intensity of the transmitted beam is measured by the detector. The transmittance is the ratio of the transmitted intensity to the original beam intensity, and the transmittance as a function of position x along the pipe diameter (see Fig. 1) is the

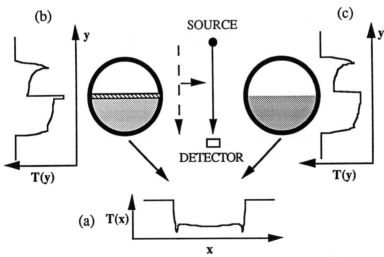

Fig. 1   Simulated x-ray projections of a pipe containing two components: a) vertical projections are the same for both segregated and mixed states; b) horizontal projection for segregated state; c) horizontal projection for mixed state.

projection. (For absorbance measurements such as CT, the projection is actually the magnitude of the natural logarithm of the transmittance, the logarithm being necessary to linearize the projection data.) A simulated 1-D projection (transmittance, T) is shown in Fig. 1(a) for the extreme cases of complete mixing and complete segregation. These projections are nearly the same, because projection removes the depth dependence of the data; therefore a thin layer of one material floating on another has approximately the same total attenuation as a well-mixed combination of the two components. (This conclusion is strictly correct only in the case of uniform sample thickness; due to the curved walls of the pipe, the projections in Fig. 1(a) actually differ by as much as 1%.) Obviously, a second projection taken at right angles to the first could easily distinguish between these two cases, as depicted in Figs. 1(b) and 1(c). In general, many projections are needed to define a unique cross section.

As discussed in Chapter 2, there are a variety of sensors that can be used to collect the projection data. For example, these sensors may be based on radiation, microwaves, light, ultrasound or acoustics, electrical capacitance, impedance (including resistance), or inductance. The electrical methods are noteworthy for their ability to obtain multiple projection data by electrical switching of their electrodes, which completely encircle the cross section to be imaged. In general, transmission techniques such as x-ray Computed Tomography require a rotation of the source/detector assembly (or else multiple stationary sources and detectors) in order to obtain the necessary data. The first part of this volume discusses several sensing methods (modalities) that are used in process tomography.

In order to complete the tomographic procedure, a cross sectional image is reconstructed from the projection data. In essence, the information contained in each pixel of the cross sectional image is distributed across the multiple projections; the task of reconstruction is therefore to gather the information from the projections in an appropriate way. The reconstruction step is defined to a large extent by the physical sensing mechanism (see Chapter 10), but in general there are several reconstruction algorithms for each modality. The most wide-spread of these algorithms, filtered backprojection, is explained by way of example in Chapter 9. The second part of this volume examines some of the other available reconstruction techniques.

A complete tomographic method consists of a modality combined with a reconstruction algorithm. Some of the tomographic methods currently used in process tomography are listed below with references to the relevant discussion in the text:

- Computed Tomography (CT) (x-ray, gamma-ray, neutron) - Chapters 17, 18, and 23
- Electrical Capacitance Tomography (ECT) - Chapters 4, 13, and 16
- Electrical Charge Tomography - Chapter 3
- Electrical Impedance Tomography (EIT) - Chapter 12
- Electrical Inductance Tomography - Chapter 8
- Electrical Resistance Tomography (ERT) - Chapters 15, 21, and 22
- Microwave Tomography - Chapter 6
- Nuclear Magnetic Resonance Imaging (NMRI, MRI) - Chapters 5 and 19
- Optical Tomography - Chapter 7
- Positron Emission Tomography (PET) - Chapters 20 and 21
- Seismic Tomography - Appendix (Abstract C.2)
- Ultrasonic Tomography - Appendix (Abstracts A.4, B.9, and D.7)

3. Applications

The motivation to develop process tomography is furnished by the tantalizing possibility of measuring previously unattainable information about the interior of industrial processes. Therefore the ultimate utility of process tomography depends on practical applications of this technology. In order to illustrate the variety of industrial applications where process tomography has been useful, a few examples are given below.

Flow imaging [8] is one of the most widespread applications of process tomography, particularly for two-component and multi-component flow measurement. By imaging the boundaries between different components, it is possible to measure the flow regime, vector velocity, and component concentrations in process vessels, reactors, and pipe lines. Two important applications are in the oil industry: monitoring the output of oil wells and measuring the water content in tankers. In addition, the study of multicomponent flow can improve the operation and design of process equipment for handling multicomponent mixtures.

Pneumatic conveying is an important (but sometimes overlooked) operation in the manufacture and use of particulate solids, powders, and flakes. The use of ECT, for example, can identify the flow regime and the degree of entrainment [9]. The flow rate of the solids can be measured more accurately than with conventional methods, improving the control and the efficiency of the manufacturing operation. Process tomography can also aid in the design of equipment to maintain the optimum flow conditions. This technology has also been used as a diagnostic tool for fluidized beds [10].

The design of process equipment determines (to an extent) how well the process performs: problems of instability or poor yield are often traceable to design flaws. Such flaws may be due to the fact that the process does not operate in the manner assumed by the designer. Tomographic techniques can give the process engineer a better understanding of the process fundamentals, which can lead to improvements in the equipment design. One example is based on the study of mixer performance using Positron Emission Particle Tracking (PEPT), which is based on the technology used for Positron Emission Tomography (PET) [11]. By placing a radioactive tracer pellet in a plowshare mixer, the trajectory of that volume of material can be recorded. The confinement of the pellet in certain regions of the mixer suggests that the mixing behavior is not uniform [12]. By comparing the trajectories obtained with a number of different mixer designs, it is possible to quantify the mixing efficiency. Thus, the best mixer for the job is chosen on the basis of its actual performance under normal operating conditions. Other process tomography methods have been used to examine the flow of material in chemical reactors.

The third section of this volume discusses several additional applications of process tomography, including the following:

- Detecting underground leaks from storage tanks - Chapter 15
- Analyzing fluidized beds - Chapter 16
- Determining the quality of mixing operations - Chapters 19 and 20
- Visualization of segregation in powders - Chapter 21

- Monitoring performance of hydrocyclones - Chapters 18 and 22
- Analyzing liquid flow distribution in trickle-bed reactors - Chapter 23

Research in these areas of application are in the forefront of this rapidly developing field, and it is hoped that this volume will elucidate the role process tomography has in a variety of industrial applications.

References

[1]   J. Radon, Berichte Verh. Sachsische Akad. Wiss., Leipzig, Math. Phys. Kl. **69:** 262-7 (1917).

[2]   G. N. Hounsfield, Brit. J. Radiol. **46:** 1016-22 (1973).

[3]   J. G. Webster, ed., Electrical Impedance Tomography (Adam Hilger, Bristol, 1990).

[4]   A. R. Crews and R. H. Bossi, Wright Laboratory Report WL-TR-91-4109 (Wright-Patterson Air Force Base, Ohio, 1992)

[5]   Y. Nagayama and A. W. Edwards, Rev. Sci. Instrum. **63:** 4757-9 (1992)

[6]   N. MacCuaig, J. P. K. Seville, W. B. Gilboy and R. Clift, Appl. Optics **24:** 4083-5 (1985).

[7]   S. M. Huang, A. B. Plaskowski, C. G. Xie, and M. S. Beck, J. Phys. E: Sci. Instrum. **22:** 173-7 (1989).

[8]   A. Plaskowski, M.S. Beck, R. Thorn, and T. Dyakowski, Imaging Industrial Flows (IOP Publishing, Bristol, 1995).

[9]   M. S. Beck, R. G. Green, and R. Thorn, J. Phys. E **20:**835-40 (1987).

[10]   G. E. Fashing and N. S. Smith, Rev. Sci. Instrum. **62:**2243-51 (1990).

[11]   D. J. Parker et al., Nucl. Instrum. Methods Phys. Res. A **348:**583-92 (1994).

[12]   C. J. Broadbent, J. Bridgwater, and D. J. Parker, in Proceedings of ECAPT '94, ed. M. S. Beck et al. (UMIST, Manchester, 1994), pp. 3-14.

Part I

Modalities

Chapter 2

The Physical Basis of Process Tomography

E. J. Morton
Department of Physics
University of Surrey
Guildford GU2 5XH U.K.

S. J. R. Simons
Department of Chemical and Biochemical Engineering
University College London
Torrington Place, London WC1E 7JE U.K.

1. Introduction

A number of research groups are now working within industry and academia on the development of techniques and applications for imaging chemical processes. Much of this work has been directed towards the instrumentation required to obtain useful process images. However, the emphasis is gradually turning towards the use of such instrumentation for process development and process monitoring. So far, very little work has been conducted on integrating imaging systems directly into process control systems.

It is the aim of this paper to describe some areas in which tomographic inspection may be relevant, and secondly to describe the physical phenomena which govern the interaction of imaging systems with a particular process. Using this information, it is then possible to outline a set of simple criterion which the practicing engineer may use to quickly determine if there is a likely tomographic solution to his particular needs. Finally, some predictions are made regarding the most likely role of process tomography in the future.

2. Industrial applications

It is not possible to describe all possible situations in which a tomographic image may be useful in the process industries, but a list of some of the more commonly identified areas is given for a number of industries in Table 1.

Energy	Analysis of pipelines, separators, fluidisers, storage tanks, furnaces, boilers, turbines, environmental contamination.
Food	Evaluation of consistency, water content, foreign bodies.
Chemicals	Characterisation of mixers, fluidisers, separators, conveyors and heat exchangers.
Minerals	Study of composition and structure. Methods for separation.

Table 1 Some industrial applications relevant to process tomography

Alternatively, rather than categorising by industry, it is interesting to list applications as a function of process dimension D, as presented in Table 2. Here D could represent a vessel diameter, for example. It is seen that most of these applications relate to process diagnostics and could therefore, in principle, be incorporated into control systems. The problem is now to understand how the physical principles which constrain a particular imaging technique can be exploited to get the best possible image based data for each application area.

3. Tomographic imaging techniques

There are a wide range of imaging techniques which may be considered for process imaging. These techniques can be categorised into three main areas: (1) those based on electrical measurements, (2) those based on acoustic signals, and (3) those based on electromagnetic and particulate radiation. In the following sections, the underlying principles of each technique are examined, and their practical importance for process imaging assessed.

D < 0.05m	Growth of fibres, foams, composites. Structural studies of filters, minerals, agglomerates, sediments, combustion. Flow in pipework, valves.
0.05m < D < 1.0m	Study of multi phase components in mixers, fluidisers, separators, risers. Flow in pipelines, pipework, conveyors. Integrity of vessels, linings.
D > 1.0m	Study of large scale risers, FCC's, adsorbtion beds, mixers, plants. Evaluation of sediment buildup, uniformity of packing or mixing, environmental contamination.

Table 2 Typical applications as a function of process dimension, D

3.1 Electrical methods

Electrical methods include capacitance, impedance and inductance tomography and magnetic resonance imaging. The basic layout for a capacitance based imaging system is shown in Fig. 1a. Here, an alternating voltage is applied to an electrode, and the capacitance to each of the other electrodes is measured. (This is possible since i = Cdv/dt ; we know dv/dt and we can measure i.) Such measurements are made very quickly (on the order of milliseconds), so there is the potential for high frame rate imaging. In the ideal world, the electrodes would be placed on the outside wall of the vessel to be imaged, and in this case, we can draw the equivalent circuit as shown in

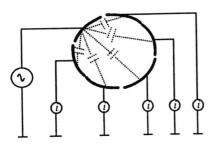

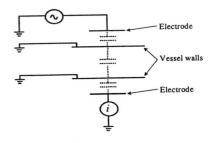

Fig. 1a Schematic illustration of a capacitance tomography system.

Fig. 1b Equivalent circuit of a capacitance system attached to the external surface of a conducting vessel.

Fig. 1b. It is seen that if the vessel wall is conducting (e.g. it is a metal wall), then the signal due to the vessel contents is shorted out. Therefore, the electrodes need either to be placed on a vessel with non-conductive walls, or inside in direct contact with the vessel contents. Most capacitance tomography to date has utilised external electrodes attached to perspex pipework.

Electrical impedance systems require a direct electrical connection between a set of electrodes and the vessel contents, with the equivalent circuit as shown in Fig. 2a. In this case, Z_v is the impedance of the vessel contents, Z_w is the impedance of the vessel wall and i_{sig} is the applied current. Thus, the currents flowing through the vessel contents, i_v, and wall, i_w, may be written as

$$i_v = \frac{Z_w}{Z_w + Z_v} i_{sig} \qquad i_w = \frac{Z_v}{Z_w + Z_v} i_{sig}$$

When the vessel wall is made of a conductive material, then $Z_w \ll Z_v$, so $i_w \approx i_{sig}$ and virtually no signal is derived from the vessel contents. Thus, we must conclude that the vessel wall must be non-conductive for this technique to be applicable. Referring to Fig. 2b, it is seen that the current flow through the vessel will follow the path of least resistance. This means that the current path between pairs of electrodes will be dependent on the composition of the vessel contents, and thus the reconstruction problem can become rather complex.

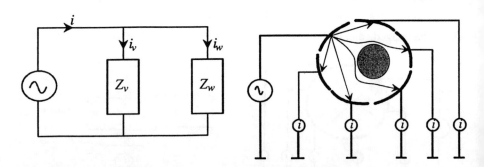

Fig. 2a Equivalent circuit of an impedance tomography system

Fig. 2b Schematic illustration of current flow through the vessel.

Similar arguments apply to inductance imaging and eddy current imaging, and again these techniques are not compatible with a metal vessel wall.

Of great interest is magnetic resonance imaging, MRI. This method uses a combination of RF and static magnetic fields to produce excellent images of certain chemical species, most notably water. Unfortunately, the technique does not cope well with conductive materials (since they shield the RF field and distort the magnetic field due to the generation of eddy currents), nor is it particularly sensitive at imaging most solid materials. However, the method can find a number of applications in areas such as diffusion in polymers and measuring water content in foods.

3.2 *Acoustic methods*

Acoustic methods derive their signal from the partial reflection of a pressure wave at a boundary between two materials of different acoustic impedance, as illustrated diagrammatically in Fig. 3a. Here, the reflection coefficient, R, may be written as

$$R = \frac{(Z_1 - Z_2)}{(Z_1 + Z_2)}$$

where Z_1 = acoustic impedance of the medium in which the acoustic wave is travelling, and Z_2 = acoustic impedance of the medium at the boundary. Suppose that the ultrasound transducer is placed on the external surface of the vessel, and that the signal is intended to propagate into the vessel contents, as shown in Fig. 3b. Here Z_1 and Z_2 are quite different, and as little as 0.1% of the signal may propagate into the vessel from

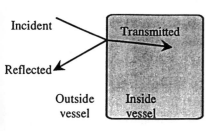

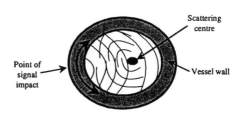

Fig. 3a Scattering of an acoustic wave at a boundary.

Fig. 3b Propagation of acoustic signals within a vessel.

the wall. As the signal propagates through the vessel, it will scatter from boundaries of different impedance, as shown in Fig. 3b. Thus the resulting signal is extremely complex to restore back into a tomographic image.

Due to this loss of transmitted power at the boundary, it is typically necessary to place the transducer in contact with the vessel contents. Thus, the technique is usually invasive to the vessel. As an alternative, it is possible to listen to the signals emanating form the vessel with no external stimulus. This is known as acoustic emission imaging, but the principles, and problems, remain the same as for more conventional ultrasound imaging. It is important to note that attenuation of the acoustic signal increases with frequency; therefore ultrasound signals can be strongly attenuated in traversing relatively small vessels.

3.3 *Electromagnetic radiation and particulate methods*

Electromagnetic radiation methods include optical, γ-ray and X-ray imaging. Obviously, optical methods may only be used for transparent objects, but problems of refraction can give rise to complex reconstruction algorithms. However, successful images have been obtained of combustion chambers and detergent foams. More conventionally, γ-ray and X-ray systems are capable of producing high quality images in a range of situations. However, Fig. 4a shows that attenuation of the radiation signal restricts maximum vessel diameters to around 1m, while Fig. 4b indicates that

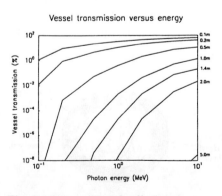

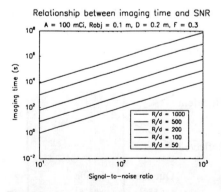

Fig. 4a Attenuation of radiation as a function of vessel diameter (0.1 m to 5.0 m diameters shown here).

Fig. 4b Variation in imaging time as a function of spatial resolution and contrast resolution.

imaging times can be long if both high spatial resolution (large R/d) and good contrast resolution (high signal-to-noise) are required from the same scan. When these requirements are relaxed, however, relatively fast imaging times can become possible under certain situations. Although radiation sources require operator protection, the technique may be used non-invasively with metal walled vessels, thus allowing a range of problems to be addressed which may not be studied so easily using other methods. In Fig. 4b, R = vessel radius, d = image resolution, A = source activity, D = source to detector distance and F = fraction of X- or (γ-radiation transmitted through the vessel.

The most widely known particulate imaging method is that of positron emission tomography (PET). This technique has recently been extended into positron emission particle tracking (PEPT) which is proving to be a valuable tool in the area of non-invasive study of rapidly changing systems, such as mixers and fluidisers, which may or may not have a metal wall. Due to attenuation of the 511 keV γ-rays produced during the annihilation of the positron, the technique is limited to working at a vessel diameter of around 30 cm. Particle position update times for the PEPT technique can be as low as a few milliseconds, while full 3D PET scans can take many hours.

Neutrons have been used successfully for many one-dimensional imaging problems in both transmission and reflection geometry. Their use for tomographic imaging is restricted due to problems of operator protection. However, thermal neutrons are extremely useful for determining the presence of low-Z materials (e.g. oil and corrosion products) in the presence of high-Z materials (e.g. steel), and consequently they receive considerable interest in the field of non-destructive testing.

3.4 *New imaging methods*

Of significant interest to the process industry are techniques for imaging the contents of large vessels (D > 1m). This is not surprising since a large fraction of the world's chemicals are produced in such vessels! Since most large vessels tend to be made of metals, and often operate at high temperatures and pressures, it is obvious that none of the standard techniques are able to satisfy the non-invasive requirements posed by large vessel imaging.

Therefore, we propose the new technique of cosmic ray muon tomography [1]. Our calculations indicate that naturally occurring cosmic ray muons may be harnessed to provide relatively detailed images of large vessels over a period of hours to days, depending on the quality of the image required. The technique is summarised in Fig. 5a, where it is shown that we need to track the direction and time at which each muon enters and exits the vessel. Since muons interact almost exclusively with atomic electrons, the degree of scattering experienced by the muon is indicative of the integral density along its path length. Therefore, we have the prospect of quantitative physical density imaging in two or three dimensions. A simulated muon image of a 10m diameter vessel with a 24 hour imaging time is shown in Fig. 5b. We believe that the technique could have a profound impact in process diagnostics, for example in helping to plan routine maintenance, plotting the packing density in adsorbtion beds, locating slippage of trays in FCC's etc.

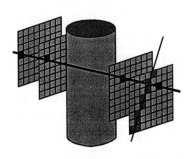
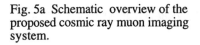
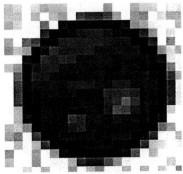

Fig. 5a Schematic overview of the proposed cosmic ray muon imaging system.

Fig. 5b Simulated 10m diameter vessel image after a 24-hour integration period.

4. Applications and techniques

To reconcile the applicability of a given imaging technique with the application areas stated in section 2 above, it is useful to study Table 3 which outlines some important characteristics of possible process applications, and their impact on the selection of imaging systems.

Vessel wall construction	Metal walls usually preclude the use of electrical, ultrasound and optical methods.
Vessel dimension	Vessels dimensions greater than 1 m cannot usually be imaged using ionising radiation.
Rate of change of vessel contents	Rapidly changing vessel contents implies a requirement for high speed imaging. This usually necessitates the use of electrical methods.
Operating temperature and pressure	If there are wide variations in operating temperature, this usually precludes the use of ultrasound methods, except when ultrasound is used as a temperature probe. High pressures usually mean non-invasive imaging which may preclude the use of electrical, optical and ultrasound methods.
Temporal and spatial resolution	Usually, temporal resolution is a tradeoff against spatial resolution (e.g. ionising radiation methods).
Quantification and spatial accuracy	Ionising radiation images are typically quantitative and spatially accurate. For electrical, optical and ultrasound methods, the reconstruction algorithm depends on the object itself, so quantification and spatial accuracy are necessarily compromised.

Table 3 Summary of the effect of process parameters on the selection of techniques

5. Conclusions

This paper has described a number of problems for which tomographic solutions may be sought, and has overviewed the limitations associated with the instrumentation which exists to provide the relevant images. However, to exploit the potential for these techniques, it is necessary to consider carefully the statements summarised in table 3 together with the more detailed analyses conducted in section 3 above. To aid this analysis, it seems that one can categorise the application areas as described in Table 2 into a set of generic areas:

STRUCTURAL ANALYSIS OF PRODUCTS/COMPONENTS

FLOW PROFILES

MIXING QUALITY

REACTOR QUALITY ASSURANCE

By describing such a set of generic areas, one can start to suggest where the most likely impact of tomographic imaging is likely to be.

The analysis of material microstructure is well suited to techniques such as MRI and high resolution X-ray imaging, which can provide excellent spatial resolution (~10 mm), good quantification, and high contrast. However, both techniques require relatively long imaging times (minutes to days), and so are suited to off-line imaging for process development and/or quality control. It is likely that these complimentary techniques will find key niche roles in this area. Detailed structural analysis of larger objects (> 10 cm diameter) can be quite problematic, unless spatial resolution at the level of > 100 mm can be tolerated. However, this is usually larger than the dimension needed to obtain useful information, so structural analysis of larger samples may not be so productive.

Analysis of flow profiles is an area where electrical techniques are already beginning to prove their value in the industrial context. Due to the problems introduced by conductive vessel walls, the requirement to insert electrodes in contact with the vessel contents, and the consequent requirement for modification of the process vessel itself, it is likely that these techniques will remain used primarily at pilot scale dimensions, with few systems being retrofit to existing full scale plant until the potential for the technique has been investigated more thoroughly. It is possible that radiation scattering techniques (although not tomographic) will prove valuable for undersea pipeline imaging (where radiation protection issues are not so critical). The use of such a method for the early detection of water slugs in a gas pipeline, for example, could have a significant impact on the efficiency of land based processing plant.

Mixing is a widely used technique which is not easily addressed using tomographic techniques due to the continual movement implicit in the process and the relatively poor contrast of many of the feedstocks (e.g. liquid-liquid or solid-solid systems). However, the positron particle tracking technique looks very promising for process development, although is not an obvious candidate for on-line production imaging. Although electrical techniques have been used to study small bench-top mixers, it is not clear that the technique will scale well to larger process scale mixers due to the amount of moving metalwork implicit in such a mixer.

Reactor quality assurance covers a range of applications ranging including analysis of the extent of fluidisation in a vessel to the integrity of a gas storage cylinder.

Usually, these applications require good quantification to observe, for example, the presence of escape channels in a packed adsorbtion bed, the integrity of vessel lagging or the buildup of scale around the vessel wall. These measurements are typically conducted on static objects, and thus are best suited to the quantitative and spatially accurate ionising radiation based methods, such as gamma-ray tomography. Since these systems are non-invasive to the vessel, they can be retrofit to existing vessels, and thus truly work at the process scale. However, many tradeoffs must be analysed for every case before it is possible to decide whether a particular geometry will be feasible. Other techniques such as eddy-current imaging and ultrasonic imaging are ideal for locating hair-line cracks and other defects in metal vessel walls, valves and pipework.

We conclude, therefore, that the most likely applications of process tomography lie at the process development stage, with those remaining applications mostly addressing process diagnostics. It will be interesting to see if these predictions become true!

References

[1]   *Editor's note: This concept is based in part on conversations with D. M. Scott, who suggested cosmic rays as a source of muons (private communication, March 24-25, 1994). A similar idea has been used to search for hidden chambers in the Second Pyramid of Giza; see L. W. Alvarez et al., Science 167 832-839 (1970).*

Chapter 3

Electrodynamic Sensors for Process Tomography

R. G. Green, J. Cottam, K. Evans, A. Goude, C. S. Johnson, A. Meehan, B. Naylor
School of Engineering Information Technology
Sheffield Hallam University, Sheffield S1 1WB U.K.

M. Henry
Department of Chemical Engineering
University of Bradford, Bradford BD7 1DP U.K.

M. F. Rahmat
Department of Control Engineering, Faculty of Electrical Engineering
Universiti Teknologi Malaysia, Jalan Semarak, 54100 Kuala Lumpur, Malaysia

1. Introduction

Transducers which sense the electrostatic charge carried by dry solids have applications in determining the velocity of conveyed materials and the solids volume flow rate in pneumatic conveyors [1]. The measurement is based on charge being induced onto the sensor as the charged particles flow past. The transducer is robust, low cost and has potential for applications in process tomography. In process tomography several identical transducers provide measurements which are then used to reconstruct dynamic images of the movement of material within the process. The first part of this chapter investigates the relationships between sensor size, sensor sensitivity and the frequency bandwidth of the transducer signals. The second part discusses the application of electrodynamic sensors to tomographic imaging.

2. Sensor theory

The theoretical relationships between electrode size, sensor sensitivity, and the frequency bandwidth of the induced signal due to an impulsive input are derived. These models are tested using a device where the velocity and size of the moving charged particle can be controlled and in experiments using flowing, dry sand.

2.1. Electrode sensitivity

The electrode sensitivity is modelled by considering the effect of a single charged particle, q, as it moves vertically downwards at a constant velocity, v. Then for the single charged particle, assumed to be a point charge of value q, the field uniformly radial

$$E = \frac{q}{4\pi r_i^2 \varepsilon_0}$$ (1)

This point charge induces a potential onto the surface of the small, fl[?] electrode used to sense the change in potential at a point on the wall of a no[?] conducting or dielectric pipe. It is assumed that there are no other interacting fields o[?] the electrode since there is no surface charge on the pipe wall. For a given sensor, th[?] cross-sectional area is πr_e^2 which is considered normal to the flux (figure 1). So th[?] proportion of flux passing through the sensor due to the charged particle at a distanc[?] r_i from it is

$$\frac{\pi r_e^2}{4\pi r_i^2}$$ (2)

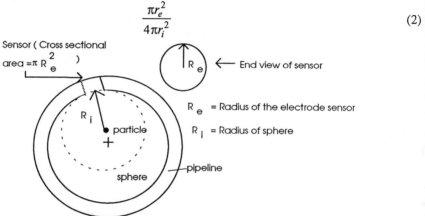

Figure 1 : Model of a charged particle in a sensing volume

The charge, Q_e, induced in the sensor is proportional to q. Hence,

$$Q_e = \frac{kqr_e^2}{r_i^2}$$ (3)

This charge is stored on a capacitor (figure 4) and provides a voltage V_e given by

$$Q_e = CV_e$$ (4)

This voltage is amplified, rectified and some smoothing applied. Equation 3 suggests the amount of charge induced onto an electrode depends upon the radius of the electrode squared. The sensitivity of the sensor is defined as $\frac{Q_e}{q_i}$. This value is difficult to determine because q_i is difficult to control or measure directly and in this paper a series of sensor diameters are compared simultaneously so that the same q_i is detected by them all.

2.2. *The spatial filtering effect*

The spatial filtering effect arising from capacitance electrodes is described in a paper by Hammer and Green [2], which relates the velocity of flowing discontinuous material to the frequency bandwidth of the sensed signal. This paper extends the concept to electrodynamic sensors. Assume that a single charged particle moving past the sensor at a distance d, with a velocity v, can be considered as a pulse of charge q(t). This moving charge results in a charge being induced into the sensor. If the sensor is shielded by the surrounding earthed screen so charge is only induced into the sensor as the particle passes along its length and assuming the inverse square law applies, the induced charge can be described by a rectangular pulse of duration a/v (figure 2). The amplitude of the charge induced into the sensor is described by:

$$\delta q_i(t) = k\frac{v}{a}\int_0^\infty \frac{q(t)}{d^2}dt \qquad (5)$$

where q(t) represents the charge pulse provided by the moving particle and k is a constant of proportionality with appropriate dimensions. If the pulse duration is short compared with a/v it may be regarded as a Dirac pulse:

$$q(t) = q_o\delta(t) \qquad (6)$$

and

$$\int_0^\infty \delta(t)dt = 1 \qquad (7)$$

and q_o is the amplitude of the charge pulse.
The amplitude of the induced charge is:

$$\delta q_i = k\frac{vq_0}{ad^2} \qquad (8)$$

The transfer function of the charge response may be written

$$\delta q_i(s) = (\frac{kvq_0}{ad^2 s})(1-\exp(-\frac{as}{v})) \qquad (9)$$

where s is the Laplace operator. Hence the electrode transfer function is

$$g(s) = (\frac{kv}{ad^2 s})(1-\exp(-\frac{as}{v})) \qquad (10)$$

which may be written in the frequency domain as

$$g(j\omega) = (\frac{kv}{ad^2 jw})(1-\exp(-\frac{aj\omega}{v})) \qquad (11)$$

The effect of a and v on the modulus of equation 11 is a sync function, shown graphically in figure 3.

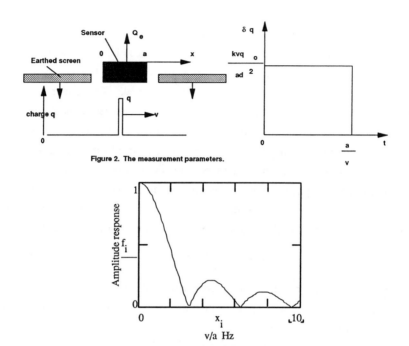

Figure 2. The measurement parameters.

Figure 3. The predicted spatial filtering effect response.

The transfer function minima occur when $\sin(\frac{\omega d}{2\upsilon}) = 0$. Therefore $\frac{\omega d}{2\upsilon} = \pi, 2\pi, 3\pi,...$

and minima occur when $\frac{\upsilon}{d} = \frac{\omega}{2\pi}, \frac{\omega}{4\pi}, \frac{\omega}{6\pi}........$ (12)

3. Electrodynamic transducer

A schematic circuit diagram of the electrodynamic transducer used in the tests is shown in figure 4.

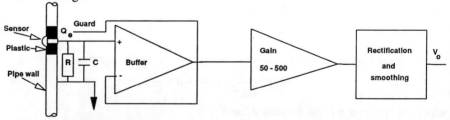

Figure 4. The transducer circuit.

The sensor consists of a metal rod, termed the electrode, which is isolated from the walls of the metal conveying pipe by an insulator, e.g. glass or plastic. This electrode has a small but variable capacitance to earth (fraction of a pico Farad), due to manufacturing tolerances. To minimise the effect of this capacitance a low value capacitor (several pico Farad) is connected in parallel with it. A resistor is connected in parallel with the capacitors to provide a charge/discharge path. The charged particles in the conveyor flow past the electrode and induce charge into it. The flow of current through the resistor due to this induced charge results in a varying voltage. This voltage is buffered by a unity gain, non inverting amplifier whose output provides a driven guard for the input circuitry and is amplified and conditioned by further circuitry.

Two experiments are presented. The first is used to determine the sensitivity of the electrode using an array of sensors and flowing sand. The second investigates the spatial filtering effect by using a charge moving past the electrode at a known velocity.

3.1. Electrode sensitivity

The sensitivity is determined by arranging a number of differently sized sensors so that sand flows past each of them in turn (figure 5). The level of charge on the flowing sand is very difficult to quantify, however since the sensors are evaluated at the same time their outputs may be compared directly with one another. The small electrode at each end of the section checks that the flowing sand does not change its characteristics as it traverses the section.

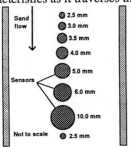

Figure 5. Arrangement of sensors for sensitivity measurement

A series of different sand flow rates are made to pass the electrodes and the resulting outputs determined. The results for each sensor are plotted graphically and a straight line regression fitted to the points; figure 6 shows a typical result for the 10 mm diameter electrode. The transducer sensitivity, consisting of the electrode sensitivity and the amplifier gain, is defined as the gradient of the graph $(mV/g\ s^{-1})$

The gain and linearity of each electronic amplifier is measured and the electrode sensitivity, defined as the transducer sensitivity divided by the electronic voltage gain, is shown in table 1 and figure 7. Figure 7 shows the result of sensitivity versus the square of the sensor diameter. The diamond points show the actual data from the experiment. Linear regression analysis was used to achieve the best straight line for all the points. The value of the correlation coefficient is 0.94. This graph supports the suggestion that the induced voltage is proportional to the square of the sensor diameter (equation 3).

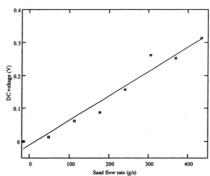

Figure 6. A typical graph for determining transducer sensitivity.

Electrode diameter (mm)	(Electrode diameter)^2 (mm^2)	Transducer sensitivity (mV/g/s)	Electronic gain	Electrode sensitivity (mV/g/s)
2.5	6.25	0.242461	162	0.00150
3	9	0.323281	160	0.00202
3.5	12.25	0.323281	154	0.00210
4	16	0.339445	156	0.00218
5	25	0.452593	159	0.00285
6	36	0.436421	156	0.00280
10	100	0.775874	145	0.00535

Table 1. Electrode sensitivity.

3.2. Spatial filtering

The spatial filtering experiment is based on the apparatus shown figure 8. A plastic ball is mounted on the wooden rod. This rod is rotated by a dc motor. The plastic ball obtains charge from an electrostatic ioniser. A charge pulse is created every time the ball passes the electrode sensor. The electrodynamic transducer senses the charge carried by the plastic ball and converts it to a voltage signal. The speed of the charged ball is varied by varying the voltage supply to the dc motor. The speed of the charged ball is calculated by measuring the circumference of the path traversed by the ball when it rotates and dividing this distance by the time between adjacent pulses.

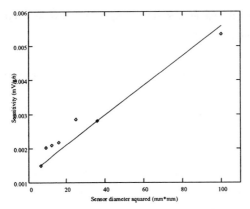

Figure 7. Electrode sensitivity versus electrode diameter squared.

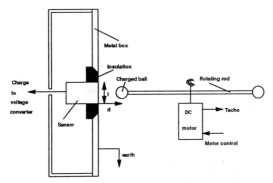

Figure 8 : Experimental set-up for spatial filtering

Figure 9 shows the spatial filtering effect for an electrodynamic sensor with a 3 mm diameter sensing electrode. The speed of the charged ball is 2.46 m/s. The power spectrum is an approximation of the sinc function, with the first cut-off frequency at 88 Hz. The spatial filtering effect is repeated for the range of electrode sizes. For a range of velocities the corresponding frequency of the first peak is determined. Equation 12 is used to calculate the predicted length of sensor corresponding to the measured frequency and velocity; this length is termed the effective length of the electrode. The mean and standard deviation of the effective length is calculated for each electrode and the bars shown in figure 10 show the mean ±3 standard deviations.

This shows the unexpected effect that the effective electrode is approximately 50 mm for the range of conditions in this experiment. Tests investigating the input network of the circuit shown in figure 4 show that the time constant of the input RC is an important factor in defining the effective electrode length. Shortening the time constant, by reducing the value of R, decreases the effective electrode length, but reduces the electronic gain of the system:

Time constant (s)	Effective electrode length (mm)
1.55×10^{-5}	42
3.60×10^{-6}	28
1.42×10^{-6}	26

An improved circuit by Shackleton [1], designed to have a wide bandwidth, is being investigated with the specific aim of minimising the effective electrode length.

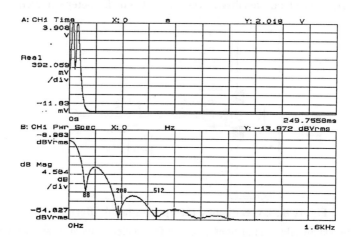

Figure 9. Spatial filtering for a 3 mm diameter sensor with v= 2.46 m/s

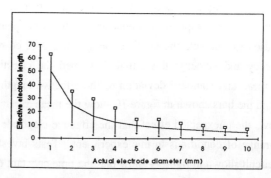

Figure 10. Effective electrode length versus actual electrode length

3.3. *Discussion on electrode tests*

The tests investigating the relationship between electrode diameter and electrode sensitivity suggest a square law as predicted by equation 3. The effective electrode length appears to be independent of the physical length of the sensor at 50 mm, but is dependent upon the design of the electronic circuit attached to the sensor. This is currently being investigated.

4. Process tomography using electrodynamic sensors.

4.1. *Introduction*

In this part of the project electrodynamic sensors and image reconstruction algorithms are being developed to produce images of velocity and concentration profiles within a cross-section of a pipe conveying the dry particulates. The basic system for process tomography is shown in figure 11. The three basic components in a process tomography system are :-(a) the sensors, (b) the data acquisition system and (c) the image reconstruction system and display. A difficulty with producing concentration images using electrodynamic sensors is that the reconstruction algorithms, which process the measured data to convert the information into a concentration profile, are dependent on the initial distribution of the solids in the sensing volume, i.e. the flow regime. If the flow regime is known, the reconstruction may be simplified and accelerated. Some flow regimes may be recognised by a suitably organised and trained neural network.

This section describes a neural network designed to classify the flow regime and select the appropriate reconstruction algorithm.

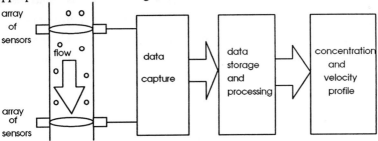

Figure 11. A process tomography system

4.2. *The measurement system*

A block diagram of the measurement system is shown in figure 12. Thirty-two sensors and transducers are positioned at equal intervals around the circumference of the pipe to provide a sensing array. This array is surrounded by an earthed metal screen, which is also connected to the pipe wall. The flowing charged particles induce charges into the sensors. These signals are conditioned, rectified and low pass filtered. These thirty-two signals are sampled and converted to eight bit format. They are then sent to both the neural network and the reconstruction algorithm.

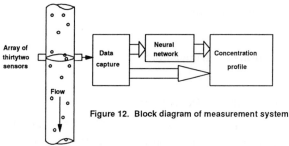

Figure 12. Block diagram of measurement system

4.3. Neural networks

The neural network consists of a three layer perceptron consisting of thirty-two input neurons, a reference neuron, eight hidden neurons and eight output neurons (figure 13). All input neurons are connected to all the hidden layer neurons. Each neuron in the hidden layer is connected to each output neuron. Both the hidden and output layer neurons use a thresholding function in the shape of a sigmoid function. The sigmoid function is represented by equation 13:

$$f(net) = \frac{1}{(1 + e^{-k(net)})} \qquad (13)$$

and has the range $0 < f(net) < 1$, where k is a positive constant that controls the spread of the function and f(net) is the Heaviside function. The system is trained using the Back Propagation Rule. This is applied by feeding appropriately processed and stored signals from the transducers for the known flow regimes to be identified into the network. The network generates a solution, which is compared with the known solution to provide an error. This error is fed back and used to modify the weightings between individual neurons. The process is repeated until the error reaches a predetermined level.

A typical data set is shown in figure 14. The input data consists of thirty-two values representing the voltages on the sensors. These voltage points are represented graphically and have been joined up to produce a voltage profile around the circumference of the pipe. A column of numbers representing the output neuron values is also included. The flow regime shown in figure 14 represents stratified flow.

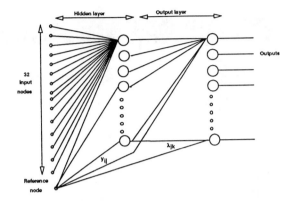

Figure 13.   The multilayer perceptron

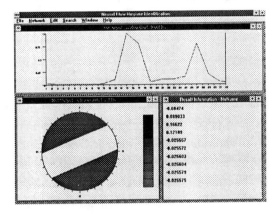

Figure 14.   Example of input and output data for the neural network

4.4. *The reconstruction algorithm*

This reconstruction algorithm is based on sensitivity distributions reported by Bidin [3] and ratio back projection. Each block of thirty-two sensor voltage values are normalised to the maximum value of the set to simplify the computation. The maximum value is stored to scale the calculated values. The pipe is considered as being divided into five radial sections and thirty-two arcs. The algorithm calculates the quantity of charge in each sector corresponding to the value on the appropriate sensor taking into account the flow profile, which is used as a weighting filter with values stored in a look up table. These calculated values are mapped onto a rectangular grid representing the cross-section of the conveyor (figure 15). The loading of all the pixels are summed to provide an estimate of the total concentration in the cross-section.

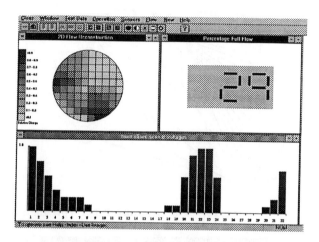

Figure 15.   Reconstructed cross section

5. Discussion

Electrical charge tomography is a relatively new technique for imaging in lightly loaded pneumatic conveyors. The successful application of the method requires careful design of the transducers (electrodes and electronics) to ensure maximum sensitivity commensurate with a bandwidth adequate with the expected range of flow velocities. Neural networks can identify several flow regimes and, after further development, may be capable of direct flow imaging [4]. However, the present work uses a purpose built reconstruction algorithm to provide tomographic images and an averaged concentration for the cross-section. Plant tests are required to verify the accuracy of the algorithms.

6. References

[1]   M. E. Shackleton, M.Phil. Thesis, University of Bradford, 1981.

[2]   E. A. Hammer and R. G. Green, J. Phys. E **16** 438-443 (1983).

[3]   A. R. Bidin, Ph.D. Thesis, Sheffield Hallam University, 1993.

[4]   A. Y. Nooralahiyan, B. S. Hoyle, and N. J. Bailey, N. J., in <u>Process Tomography - 1995: Implementation for Industrial Processes</u>, Proceedings of ECAPT '95, ed. M. S. Beck et al. (UMIST, Manchester, 1995), pp. 420-424.

Chapter 4

Sensor Design and Selection

M S Beck
Department of Electrical Engineering & Electronics
University of Manchester Institute of Science and Technology
P O Box 88, Manchester M60 1QD, UK

R A Williams
Camborne School of Mines
University of Exeter
Redruth, Cornwall TR15 3SE, UK

1. Introduction

Sensors for industrial process tomography are categorized under three operating principles: electromagnetic radiation, acoustic and measurement of electrical properties. Spatial resolution using electromagnetic radiation can be as good as 1%, but these methods have a limited range of applications due to, for example, optical opacity when using light, slow speed and radiation containment when using ionising radiation, expense when using magnetic resonance, need for operator intervention and radio-active particles when using positron emission tomography. Electrical tomographic sensors, using capacitance, conductance, inductance and microwave techniques offer a modest spatial resolution of about 10%, but they are fast, inexpensive and suitable for a wide range of vessel sizes. Acoustic sensors promise 3% spatial resolution, however, as yet there are relatively few reports confirming their suitability for *process* tomography.

The sensors named above are generally suitable for distinguishing between two phases or components in the object space being interrogated, and are referred to as *single mode* sensors. There are many processes where three or more components exist in the object space and have to be individually imaged. Examples include metallurgical ore separation, coal/shale separation, oil field pipelines and separators which contain oil, gas and water. In these situations *multi-mode* sensing systems are required.

Multi-mode tomographic imaging systems are strictly defined as those in which two or more different sensing entities are used to locate or measure different constituents in the object space. An example of dual mode tomography is taken from the oil industry. There is a need to measure the quantity of oil, gas and water in a cross section of an oil well riser. At the same time information is needed on the physical distribution of each component in the cross section in order to measure the production of the well. A specific solution uses electrical capacitance tomography for imaging and measuring the water in the oil and ultrasonic tomography for the gas (section 4).

A particular class of multi-mode systems are "inherently multi-mode systems" in which a single imaging method can be used to differentiate between different components in the object space. One inherently multi-mode system being developed for process use is based on impedance spectroscopy, in which the characteristic frequency/impedance relationship of one component (or more) in a mixture is used to image that component in the presence of several other components (section 4.1).

Electromagnetic tomography (section 4.1) is inherently multi-mode and can provide an interesting approach to multi-component imaging. This could be particularly useful for metallurgical processes and scrap recycling systems, where ferrous material could be imaged based on its magnetic permeability, and non-ferrous material could be imaged based on its eddy current loss. Impedance spectroscopy could also be incorporated in the electromagnetic system, which should extend the applicability of this totally non-contacting technique.

This chapter seeks to address principally those sensor systems that are amenable for use on-line in an industrial environment.

1.1 *Tomographic Technology*

Tomographic imaging technology involves the acquisition of measurement signals from sensors located on the periphery of an object, such as a process vessel or pipeline. This reveals information on the nature and distribution of components within the sensing zone. Ideally, it does not involve any addition or disturbance to the process. Real-time images can be obtained which measure the dynamic evolution of the parameter(s) being detected at the sensors; thus making the image data suitable for process control purposes (Figure 1). Another type of imaging technique exists, which involves the use of tracer species which are added into the process under investigation. These tracers emit an appropriate and detectable signal via sensors placed at the periphery of the vessel. The sensors can only detect and track the movements of a few individual tracer species, rather than being able to reveal a complete image of the components in the entire cross-section probed by sensors. An example of this method is positron emission tomography (PET) [1], as described elsewhere in this volume.

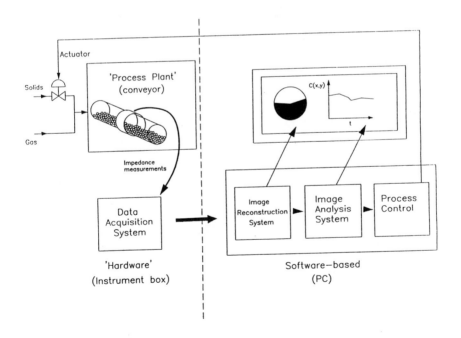

Fig. 1 Principal components in a process tomographic instrument,
in this case controlling a pneumatic conveyor

An analogous tracer technique, which utilizes specific molecules that are normally present in the process is magnetic resonance imaging (MRI). This exploits the electromagnetic properties of individual molecules in a liquid-based mixture [1].

2. Sensors for Process Tomography - Performance Envelopes

The heart of any tomographic technique is the sensor system that is deployed. The basis of any measurement is to exploit differences or contrast in the properties of the process being examined. A variety of sensing methods can be employed based on measurements of transmission, diffraction or electrical phenomena. Table 1 shows a selection of possible sensing methods and their principal attributes.

Table 1   Sensors for process tomography

Principle	Spatial Resolution (percentage of diameter of cross section)	Practical Realisation	Comment
Electromagnetic radiation	1%	Optical	Fast Optical access required
		X-ray and γ-ray	Slow radiation containment
		Positron emission	Labelled particle Not on-line
		Magnetic resonance	Fast Expensive for large vessels
Acoustic	3%	Ultrasonic	Sonic speed limitation Complex to use
Measurement of electrical properties	10 %	Capacitive Conductive Inductive	Fast Low cost Suitable for small or large vessels

As described in the introductory remarks whilst most devices employ a single type of sensor, there are a number of opportunities for multi-mode systems using two (or more) different sensing principles (section 4). The choice of sensing system will be determined largely by:

- The nature of components contained in the pipeline, vessel, reactor or material being examined (principally, whether they exist as a solid, liquid, gas or a multi-phase mixture, and if so in what proportions);

- the information sought from the process (steady-state, dynamic, resolution and sensitivity required) and its intended purpose (laboratory investigations, optimisation of equipment, process measurement or control);
- the process environment (ambient operation conditions, safety implications, ease of maintenance etc.);
- the size of the process equipment and the length-scale of the process phenomena being investigated.

3. Sensor Selection - Single Mode Tomography

Figure 2 provides guidelines for sensor selection based on the spatial resolution required by the user. Other important features such as speed, robustness etc. (Figure 3) also need to be considered. In many cases the process needs cannot be clearly and unambiguously defined, so alternative sensing methods are possible. An informed selection can be made on the basis of information contained in textbooks and reference works [1] [2]. The final choice may often be based on availability of suitable equipment tempered by engineering judgement.

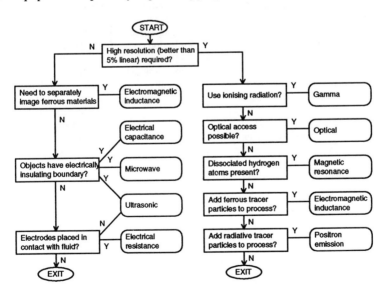

Fig. 2 Sensor selection for process tomography

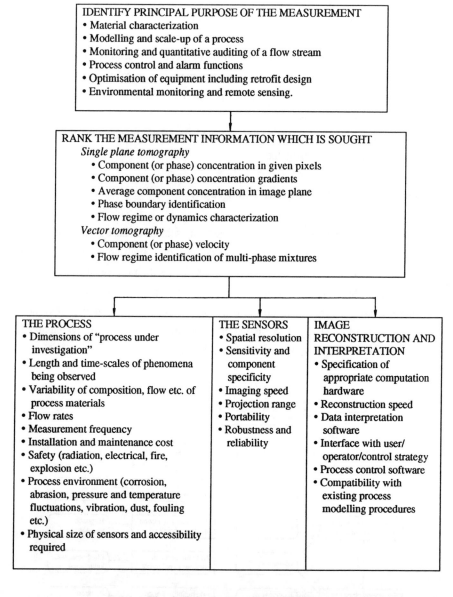

Fig. 3 Criteria for sensor selection

The first criterion is the required resolution. In many cases it will be seen that high resolution tomography can sometimes be expensive, rather slow and in some cases impose special requirements for safe operation. In contrast to this, the lower resolution methods can be relatively inexpensive, fast response and do not involve safety constraints. Therefore the process need for image resolution needs to be carefully considered. Table 2 encapsulates the interpretation of image resolution (citing the particular case of electrical tomography) in terms of the process properties that can be resolved by the tomographic system. For example, if dispersed particles have to be imaged, then a high resolution technique may be required, however in many cases it is only necessary to know the ratio of phases (i.e. void fraction in gas/liquid mixtures, volume fraction of particles, averaged over a zone in the process which is much larger than the particle size itself etc.) Thus in Table 2 it is pointed out that a tomographic system can measure the ratios of two phases within a resolved image element, even though the individual particles cannot be resolved. This information is quite often sufficient for process design and operation purposes.

Table 2 Image resolution and phase fraction measurement - the case for electrical tomography

Image Resolution (target)	1 in 20 of projection distance (diameter of process vessel) 1 in 400 of projected areas (cross-sectional area of process vessel)
Minimum size of phase boundary/particles that can be resolved	Equal to the imaging resolution above
Measurement of phases or dispersed particles too small to be resolved	Ratio of phases is measured within an imaged element even though individual particles cannot be resolved

If high resolution is required the first path in Figure 2 leads to ionising radiation. The X-ray computed tomography method is well known, but generally not suitable for on-line process use because it is bulky, uses moving parts and is relatively slow. The alternative of gamma radiation is the method of choice for real-time process tomography, because the source is very compact and with recent development in gamma sensors [3] images as fast as 10 frames per second can be obtained with a total source strength of only 250 mCi [241] Am.

For the (relatively few) processes handling transparent fluids and where optical access is possible, then optical techniques can provide high resolution images

[1,4]. An alternative high resolution imaging technique, which can be used when the process components to be imaged include dissociated hydrogen atoms (usually aqueous), is magnetic resonance imaging. [3,4] This high resolution technique is very expensive (normally requiring cryogenic cooling of the magnet) and the largest systems available are those proportioned to image the human body. Whilst it cannot operate in the presence of iron species, it does offer chemical specificity.

In some cases "tracer particle imaging" is acceptable, by which the movement of one or of several labelled tracer particles is imaged during passage through the process. Such methods (e.g. positron emission) are limited to situations where suitable neutrally buoyant particles can be obtained, where operators are available to inject the particles and where a time of, say, five times the major time constant of the process is available for collecting the image information. Generally these techniques are invaluable to verify design and scale-up of equipment, but less attractive for routine use in manufacturing plant.

The other major direction in Fig. 2 is for imaging where a resolution of better than 5% (linear) is not required, this corresponding to an area resolution of not better than 0.25%. The first question concerns the need to separately image ferrous materials, it is appropriate to the increasing number of processes handling recycled products and leads to considering the use of magnetic inductance tomography (section 4.1).

The next question concerns the electrical nature of the object space. If the object has an electrically insulating boundary (e.g. gas/liquid systems, insulating liquids etc.) then electrical capacitance tomography is becoming a well established technique for this situation. Microwave tomography is a close variant to the lower frequency capacitance techniques for process imaging, although it is probably more expensive and there are relatively few published accounts of using microwave methods on processes [1]. Ultrasonic tomography is an alternative, measuring the density properties of distributed phases rather than their electrical properties [1]. Ultrasonic techniques, although appealing at first sight, can have problems due to spurious reflections and diffraction effects and may therefore require a high degree of engineering design for any particular application.

When the process does not have an electrically insulating boundary, and when electrodes may be placed in contact with the process fluid, then electrical resistance tomography is an attractive proposition, with an extensive track record for medical applications and ever increasing use for process measurement. If electrodes cannot be placed in contact with the fluid, for reasons of pressure integrity, fouling of the electrode surface etc. then electromagnetic induction tomography (which is still at an early stage of development) could be operated in a mode whereby the eddy current loss of material in the object space is imaged, thus making it a possible future alternative to electrical resistance tomography [1].

4. Sensor Selection - Multi-mode tomography

A multi-modality tomographic system can use two or more different sensing entities (e.g. two selected from Table 1) to locate or measure different constituents in the object space. Other "multi-modality" types of measurements are common in instrumentation, for example optical spectroscopy can be used to measure several chemical species which are present along the path of a light beam, by selecting the different absorption spectra which are appropriate to the specific species.

One example of using dual-modality systems occurs in medical tomography where body imaging using X-ray computed tomography clearly images the bone structure, but is not sufficiently sensitive to differentiate between healthy and diseased soft tissue. On the other hand, magnetic resonance imaging can locate diseased tissue within other soft tissue but is not sensitive to bony structure. In cases where the surgeon wishes to know the exact position of diseased tissue relative to bone structure, both X-ray CT and MRI images are used together. Here one of the major problems in dual modality imaging occurs, both images are geometrically distorted due to the imprecise knowledge of the sensing field geometry, limitations in the construction of sensors, beam bending etc. Hence the two tomographic images do not register exactly and the relative location of the bony structure and diseased tissue cannot be relied on. In this case *image registration* can be improved by the skill of the observer who looks for anatomical features which are detected by both of the imaging modalities, who can then use this information to make appropriate adjustments in registration. Alternatively, computer aided image registration should be a feasible method of improving image registration.

The problems of image registration become greater when electrical sensors are used for tomographic imaging, because electrical field equipotentials may be severely distorted by variations in the electrical properties of the object space, with consequential distortion of the image and difficulties in image registration. This problem can sometimes be less important for some process applications, because the precise location of "objects" is not required. A more normal requirement is for information on the general distribution of materials, the flow regime, or even to use the tomographic data to provide the time averaged value of some process variable.

The dual modality tomography systems in the oil industry, discussed in section 1, exemplifies a common process measurement problem where there is a need to quantify the composition in a cross section, and at the same time to seek information on the flow regime (in this case the physical distribution of the gas and water in the cross section). From these data the productivity of the well (quantity of oil, gas and water produced) and useful information to understand the multiphase transport and separation process is obtained. One solution mentioned was to use electrical capacitance tomography for imaging and measuring the water distribution (water has approximately 40 times the permittivity of oil) [1]. The gas distribution is then determined by a system which is responsive to the large density difference between gas liquid. However, two alternative tomographic systems could be used for detecting the density difference, the alternatives being gamma tomography or ultrasonic tomography.

4.1 *Inherently Multi-modality Systems*

An inherently multi-modality system uses a single imaging method which can differentiate between different species in the object space. Thus all the measured information is available using the same measurement field and image registration is an inherent feature of the method.

Electrical tomography systems are in certain cases the most attractive for real-time imaging of industrial processes because of their inherent simplicity, rugged construction and high speed capability. During recent years work has started on exploring the potential of impedance spectroscopy and dielectric spectroscopy to increase the component specificity of electrical tomography systems. For instance, the notion of using a multi-frequency electrical impedance tomography system has been explored involving taking image readings at two different frequencies, in order to image a slowly varying or static phenomenon, when using an instrument which was not calibrated for the initial state of the object space [5]. Although not actually involving species identification, the potential of the method has been extended to this area. Other investigations of the use of impedance spectroscopy for differentiating between different materials are under active development [3]. This appears likely to lead to a system which could be incorporated within an electrical impedance tomography system to enable component specificity to be obtained provided that the impedance spectra characteristics can be attributed unambiguously to component properties.

Electromagnetic (inductive) tomography systems (described in more detail elsewhere in this volume) are capable of distinguishing between ferrous materials and electrically conducting materials in the object space. This distinction occurs because electrically conducting materials involve energy absorption by eddy-current loss, which is electrically in-phase to the applied magnetic field and can be detected by a phase-sensitive demodulator measuring the field strength. On the other hand, ferrous components in the object space affect the applied field in a vectorially orthogonal way to the eddy-current effect, and can be separately identified by a phase-sensitive demodulator using an orthogonal reference signal.

5. Conclusions

Sensor selection is a multi-factorial process often giving several alternative choices. Key factors in making a final selection for use in an industrial processes environment are -

• in-house experience
• capital and ownership costs
• availability of market-proven instrumentation

The availability of market-proven instruments is probably an overriding factor because if a special instrument has to be developed or modified, both capital and ownerships costs are difficult to estimate and can escalate quickly. Few tomographic imaging systems are yet available on a "turn key" basis. As the subject advances, more manufactured instruments will become available. Therefore after considering "fitness for purpose" of candidate sensors system(s) other important attributes will include -

- robustness of sensors
- cost/ease of manufacture of sensors having specific geometry and vessel sizes
- ease of calibration, for example can the range be altered without recalibrating the sensors
- user friendliness of operator interface
- manufacturers' policy on instrument modifications (continuous improvements will take place in these early years) and forward/backward compatibility of instrumentation subsystems.

References

[1]   Williams, R.A. and Beck, M.S. (Eds), (1995) Process Tomography - Principles, Techniques and Applications, Butterworth-Heinemann, Oxford.

[2]   Plaskowski, A., Beck, M.S., Thorn, R. and Dyakowski, T (1995) Imaging Industrial Flows, IOP Press, Bristol.

[3]   Process Tomography - Implementation in Industrial Processes, Proceedings of ECAPT'95 (Bergen), UMIST (Manchester), 1955 p. 161.

[4]   Process Tomography: Special Issue of Chem. Eng.J. (R.A. Williams, Ed.), 56 (1995) p. 83 - 192.

[5]   Riu, P, Rosell, J and Pallas-Areny, R., (1993) Multifrequency Electrical Impedance Tomography as an Alternative to Absolute Imaging, in "Tomographic Techniques for Process Design & Operation", Computational Mechanics Publications pp. 53-62.

Chapter 5

Magnetic Resonance Velocimetry

S. J. Gibbs, B. Newling, and L. D. Hall
Herchel Smith Laboratory for Medicinal Chemistry
University of Cambridge School of Clinical Medicine
University Forvie Site, Robinson Way, Cambridge, CB2 2PZ, UK

D. E. Haycock, W. J. Frith, and S. Ablett
Unilever Research Laboratories — Colworth House
Sharnbrook, Bedfordshire, MK44 1LQ U.K.

1. Introduction

Magnetic resonance (MR) techniques offer a uniquely powerful means of quantitatively probing the dynamics of a wide variety of phenomena including molecular tumbling and rearrangements, chemical reactions, translational diffusion, and flow. One important feature stems from the fact that many systems which are optically opaque are transparent at radio frequencies; hence, by combining MR imaging (MRI) techniques with MR flow sensitivity, precision velocimetry of materials and geometries which are either difficult or impossible to study by conventional techniques such as hot wire or laser Doppler anemometry is now possible. Materials may include gels, polymer solutions, concentrated particulate dispersions, polymer melts, and emulsions; geometries may include designs for specialized rheometric flows, facsimiles of process equipment such as mixers, manifolds, and packed beds, and porous media.

This chapter begins with a brief introduction to the underlying theory of MR, the required instrumentation, and the flow sensitivity. These discussions are necessarily terse, but may serve as a guide to the broader literature. We do, however, attempt to convey an appreciation of the capabilities, areas of possible application, and limitations of MR velocimetry. We then turn our attention to two specific applications of MR velocimetry (MRV): **rheometry by capillary velocimetry,** and **velocimetry of multidimensional flows for validation of computational models.** We discuss in detail the application of MR capillary velocimetry to studying the rheology of polymer solutions and particulate dispersions, and we present an example of the detection of apparent wall slip by MRV. We also present MRV data for Newtonian flow in a series of cylindrical expansions and contractions and compare these data with those generated by a commercially available computational fluid dynamics (CFD) package.

2. Background

Since the initial reports of Lauterbur [1] and Mansfield and Grannel [2,3] in 1973 on nuclear magnetic resonance imaging (MRI), methods and equipment for MRI have rapidly progressed, largely because of utility for medical diagnosis. For example, it is now possible to acquire a two-dimensional NMR image of a slice consisting of a rectangular matrix of 128 by 128 picture elements (pixels) at a spatial resolution as fine as 100 μm in approximately 100 ms by echo-planar MRI [4]. Further, the imaging protocol can be tailored to discriminate quantitatively on the basis of chemical composition, physical state, or motion and low-cost, dedicated hardware is now becoming available for specialized applications. The following brief discussion introduces some concepts and terminology used throughout the remainder of this chapter, but is by no means comprehensive; several comprehensive introductions to the theory and practice of NMR and MRI are available [5,6].

2.1 Theory of Magnetic Resonance

Nuclei with non-zero spin angular momentum, for example the proton, the deuteron, and the nuclei of ^{13}C, ^{31}P, and ^{19}F, have associated with them a nuclear magnetic moment $\vec{\mu}$. When an ensemble of such nuclei is placed in a polarizing magnetic field, the magnetic moments tend to align with the field, ultimately at equilibrium with a Boltzman distribution of energies, to produce a net magnetization, M_0, in the ensemble. Because these nuclei have spin angular momentum, there is a characteristic precession frequency, the Larmor frequency, $\omega_0 = \gamma B(1 - \sigma)$, of the nuclear magnetization about the direction of the applied magnetic field, B. Here, γ is the magnetogyric ratio of the nucleus being observed, and σ is the **chemical shift** associated with the chemical environment of the nuclei being observed. Typically, γ is on the order of `MHz/Tesla` and σ is on the order of 1-100 ppm; for protons, $\gamma \approx 42.6$ MHz/Tesla and σ is on the order of 1-10 ppm. It is the chemical-shift effect, that allows discrimination between, for example, oil and water phases in MRI.

Magnetic resonance experiments employ a radio-frequency antenna structure placed nearby the volume of interest, to perturb the nuclear magnetization from the equilibrium state (via radio-frequency pulses applied to the leads of the antenna structure) and to monitor the behaviour of the nuclear magnetization after such a perturbation; the precessing magnetization induces an oscillating voltage in the antenna structure which may be digitized and analyzed to determine component frequencies and phases. Spatial information is obtained by making the magnetic field strength B depend upon spatial position and time in such a way that the acquired signal has the following form:

$$S(\vec{k}) = \int_V \rho(\vec{r}) \exp(-i\vec{k} \cdot \vec{r}) \, d\vec{r} \qquad (1)$$

where, $\vec{k} = \int \gamma \vec{g} \, dt$, $\vec{g}$ is the applied, time-dependent magnetic field gradient, and $\rho(\vec{r})$ is the local transverse magnetization as a function of the spatial coordinate $\vec{r}$. Hence, the raw MRI data may be acquired in a k-space that is truly the Fourier conjugate to the image space. This conjugate space is normally scanned in a raster-like fashion with either multiple radio-frequency excitations, as in spin-warp spin-echo [7] or FLASH [8] imaging, or a single radio-frequency excitation, as in echo-planar imaging (EPI) [4].

The acquired signal can also be made very sensitive to the dynamics of the system under study. The rate at which the nuclear magnetization returns to equilibrium after a radio-frequency perturbation (characterized by two relaxation times: T_1, the longitudinal relaxation time, and T_2 the transverse relaxation time) is sensitive to molecular motions at frequencies on the order of the Larmor frequency and to the presence of paramagnetic substances. Hence these phenomena, may be used to monitor, for example, physical phase changes and the local concentration of paramagnetic species; in combination with serial imaging, reaction kinetics, fluid flow, and interdiffusion on time scales of seconds to hours may be studied [9,10]. Further, by employing specialized sequences of radio-frequency and magnetic field gradient pulses, diffusive and coherent motion on a time scale of milliseconds and length scales of μm to mm may be measured [11-13]. These techniques are useful for making maps of fluid velocities and intradiffusion coefficients.

2.2 Instrumentation for Magnetic Resonance

We now give a cursory description of modern MRI equipment in order to convey better the scale of complexity of the apparatus involved and the spatial constraints and other limitations imposed by conventional MRI systems.

A system for performing MRI consists of the following components: a magnet for polarising the sample; a computer system for controlling radio-frequency and field-gradient pulses and the radio-frequency receiver; a computer system for data processing and display; radio-frequency and audio-frequency amplifiers; a radio-frequency probe (antenna); and gradient coils for generating the required spatial magnetic field variation. The experimental data described in this chapter were acquired with either an Oxford Resarch Systems Biospec I console and an Oxford Instruments 2 Tesla, 31 cm bore magnet or a Bruker MSL 200 console running Tomikon imaging software (version Medizin Technik GmBH, Karlsruhe, Germany) and an Oxford Magnet Technology 1 m bore 2 Tesla magnet. Custom built radio-frequency probes and gradient coils were used for each application. Experimental data were transferred to Unix workstations for reconstruction, analysis, and display.

2.3 Flow Sensitivity of Magnetic Resonance

The flow sensitivity of magnetic resonance techniques has been exploited for many years [14,15], and current practice has been recently reviewed [11-13]. These methods can be loosely categorized into magnitude and phase based techniques, which respectively exploit the magnitude and orientation of the local nuclear magnetization vector $\vec{M}$ as fluid tags which can be monitored in space and time. By imaging the local magnetization state after the creation and evolution of these tags, one can create images of local displacements and thus infer the velocity field.

An especially graphic display of complex flow fields can be created directly by so-called DANTE [16] tagged MRI, in which the magnitude of the local magnetization is nulled in orthogonal sets of planes in the volume to be be imaged. After a suitable evolution delay, during which time the nulled planes move with the local fluid velocity, the magnetization state is imaged [17-20]. If this process is repeated for two or more durations of the evolution delay, then local fluid displacements per unit time can be determined. Although rigorously tracking the positions of tags through time is not trivial in practice, manual examination of the series of tagged images assists in developing a qualitative appreciation of the general features of the velocity field in the region of interest.

More quantitative studies of the velocity field can be made by phase-based velocity sensitization methods, which encode in the phase of the local nuclear magnetization the displacement over a time interval Δ [12]. The measured signal $A(\vec{r})$ from a voxel then has a dependency upon translational motion given by

$$A(\vec{r}) \approx \int_V A_0(\vec{r}) \exp[\Delta(i\vec{v}(\vec{r}) \cdot \vec{k} - \vec{k} \cdot \mathbf{D}(\vec{r}) \cdot \vec{k})] \, d\vec{r} \qquad (2)$$

where $A_0(\vec{r})$ is a function of the local proton density and relaxation times, $\vec{v}(\vec{r})$ is the local fluid velocity, $\mathbf{D}(\vec{r})$ is the local intradiffusion tensor, $\vec{k}$ is a function of the magnitude and duration of phase encoding magnetic field gradient pulses used for motion encoding, and the integral is over the voxel volume. Hence, by performing experiments for several values of $\vec{k}$, the average velocities for each voxel may be determined. Modern frequency analysis methods are proving useful for this purpose [21].

3. Applications

3.1 Fluid Rheology Studied by MRI Capillary Velocimetry

The complex rheology of heterogeneous fluids such as concentrated particulate dispersions, emulsions, and foams coupled with the optical opacity of many such systems make them suitable for study with current magnetic resonance velocimetric techniques. Of particular interest are the phenomena of apparent wall slip, shear polarization, and extensional effects. Magnetic resonance methods potentially allow the measurement of velocity fields with a spatial resolution of some tens of microns and velocity resolution on the order of 10 μm/s. Time resolution currently limits most studies to steady systems, but snapshot measurements of velocities on a time scale of hundreds of milliseconds are possible in specialized situations.

Widespread availability of NMR imaging hardware is now allowing the implementation of advanced NMR velocimetric methods for studying fundamental rheology [20,22-27]. Work to date has included studies of polymer rheology in capillary [22] and more complex [23] geometries, studies of pastes and suspensions in capillary and Couette flow [24-26], flow in porous media, thermal convection, and turbulence[20].

NMR velocimetric imaging of rheometric flows, or **NMR rheometry**, has been demonstrated for Couette and Poiseuille flows [22,24-26]. In these applications, assumptions of no slip at the solid surfaces and uniform shear in the Couette device may be directly checked by velocimetric imaging. Also, the resulting velocity fields may be processed together with information concerning the wall shear stress in order to determine the intrinsic viscosity of the fluid as a function of the **observed** shear rates.

We present results here for a Newtonian sucrose solution, shear-thinning polymer solutions, and a particulate gel system. For the sucrose solution, Newtonian behavior is confirmed by NMR rheometry, and the Newtonian viscosity thus determined agrees well that that determined by cone-and-plate rheometry. Results for a 0.2% aqueous xanthan gum solution are consistent with cone-and-plate rheometry, and show little evidence of apparent wall slip. The particulate gel system shows large apparent slip velocities at the capillary wall. Potential for further work for characterization of slip effects, shear polarization, and extensional effects are discussed.

The experimental apparatus for the capillary rheometry work described here comprises a 2 Tesla superconducting magnet and 4 mm id 1 m in length precision bore glass capillary through which the fluid under study is pumped from a pressure reservoir via a peristaltic pump. Flow encoded images were acquired by a gradient echo technique [5,6] and flow velocities were estimated by Bayesian frequency analysis [21]. Two dimensional velocity maps were then processed to obtain radial velocity profiles [22]. For fully developed Poiseuille flow, radial velocity profiles for different average velocities and solutions may be differentiated to obtain estimates of the dependence of viscosity upon shear rate;

$$\eta = \alpha r (\frac{dv}{dr})^{-1} = \alpha r \dot{\gamma}^{-1} \tag{3}$$

where the constant of proportionality α is one half the pressure drop per unit length of tubing. Here, v is the fluid velocity, r is the radial coordinate in the tube, and $\eta(\dot{\gamma})$ is the shear-rate dependent fluid viscosity.

We now consider in more detail some examples of rheometric applications of MRV. Figure 1 shows the parabolic velocity profile for flow of an aqueous sucrose

Figure 1: Velocity pro-
file for 50.4% aqueous sucrose in 4mm ID glass capillary. Points correspond
to experimental measure-
ments, and error bars correspond to standard de-
viations for 50 points in
small radial neighborhood
around the average radial
position. Line corresponds
to expected parabolic ve-
locity profile for fully developed Newtonian flow.

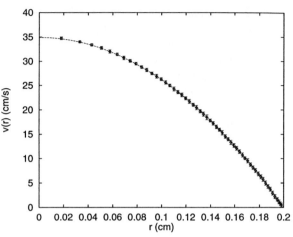

solution through the 4 mm ID glass tube. The experimental points are in excellent
agreement with the parabola expected for fully developed Poiseuille flow of a
Newtonian fluid. Data like these were also obtained for 0.2% aqueous xanthan
gum and used to calculate the shear-rate dependence of viscosity as described
in equation (3). A comparison of these data with the results of cone-and-plate
rheometry is shown in Fig. 2; both sets of data indicate that the shear-rate
dependence of viscosity for 0.2% aqueous xanthan gum is very nearly power-law.
Figure 3 shows a velocity profile obtained for a high volume fraction dispersion of
gel particles (50-100 micron). This particulate system exhibits so-called *apparent
wall slip*; the velocity profile does not intercept zero velocity at the capillary wall.
A likely explanation is that the gel particles are excluded from the wall region and
that there is thus a thin layer of fluid near the wall with reduced viscosity; because
of its reduced viscosity as compared with the bulk fluid, this thin, so-called *slip
layer* sustains a high shear rate thus causing an apparent non-zero fluid velocity
at the wall.

3.2 Comparisons of MR Velocimetry and CFD for Multidimensional Flows

Comparisons of MRV and CFD results are useful for validating underlying
CFD models and checking solution techniques for multidimensional flows. Of
particular interest in this context are the effects of non-Newtonian shear viscosity
and extensional viscosity. An interesting test case is shown in Fig. 4; here is

Figure 2: Comparison of cone-and-plate and NMR rheometry for 0.2% aqueous xanthan gum solution: Plot of viscosity versus shear rate. Note that the dependence is nearly linear on the log-log scale (power law behavior). The points are results from NMR rheometry and the diamonds are results from cone-and-plate rheometry.

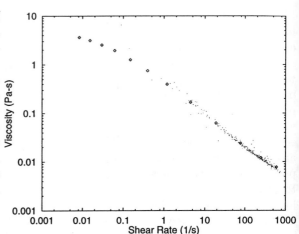

Figure 3: MR velocimetry for Poiseuille flow of a high volume fraction dispersion of gel particles. Points correspond to experimental measurements, and error bars correspond to standard deviations for 50 points in small radial neighborhood around the average radial position. The profile exhibits a flat central region reflecting the presence of a *yield stress* and pronounced apparent wall slip.

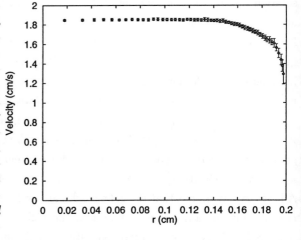

shown the geometry of an expansion-contraction-expansion-contraction (ECEC) pipe system. In this system, extensional flow effects are potentially significant for non-Newtonian fluids; we consider in the following discussion results of MRV and CFD for Newtonian fluids.

A qualitative appreciation of the flow field present in the (ECEC) system may be attained by so-called DANTE tagged MRI (as described above). In this scheme, magnetization in selected orthogonal planes orthogonal also to the imag-

ng plane is nulled by frequency-selective radio-frequency excitation in the presence of magnetic field gradient pulses. The images in Fig. 4 were acquired after an
ncremented delay from the end of the tagging procedure. The fluid recirculation
n the expansions and the large difference between the recirculation velocities and
the central forward velocity are readily apparent from inspection of these images;
also differences between the flow in the first and second expansions are evident.

A more detailed view of the velocity field may be obtained by a phase sensitive velocity encoding technique coupled with a Bayesian frequency analysis for
estimation of the local velocities and fitting (eq. (2)) errors. Figure 5 shows such
results for the axial component of velocity in the ECEC system. Results here were
actually obtained by three methods: flow encoded echo planar imaging (EPI); flow
encoded gradient echo imaging (FLASH); and simulation by a commercial CFD
package (FIDAP, Fluid Dynamics International). The EPI and FLASH MRV
techniques employed are rapid, three-dimensional imaging techniques; imaging
times for each 64×64×64 pixel flow encoded image were approximately five minutes and thirty minutes respectively. The EPI imaging results, although obtained
more rapidly, are corrupted because of the long echo times (approximately 100ms)
employed; during the long NMR transient, fast moving fluid in the central channel
moves several pixels and is not reliably registered in the flow-encoded EPI images.
The FLASH technique employs shorter NMR transients (approximately 20 ms)
and yields axial velocities which compare more favorably with the CFD results.
It is important to note, however, that the finite NMR transient time and motion
encoding intervals will always cause some spatial misregistration of the velocity
field and temporal averaging of the local fluid velocities; these effects are largest
for systems with fast flow and large fluid accelerations but may be ameliorated
by using specially designed NMR pulse sequences [28,29].

4. Conclusions

Magnetic resonance velocimetry has great potential for improving our understanding of the rheological behavior of complex fluids in processing equipment.
We have demonstrated capabilities of MRV for one-dimensional capillary flow and
for multidimensional flows. Capillary MRV is useful for rheometry of opaque fluids
and for studying slip phenomena. Single velocimetric measurements can provide
data on the shear-rate dependence of fluid viscosity over the complete range of
shear rates present in the capillary flow. Velocimetry of multidimensional flows

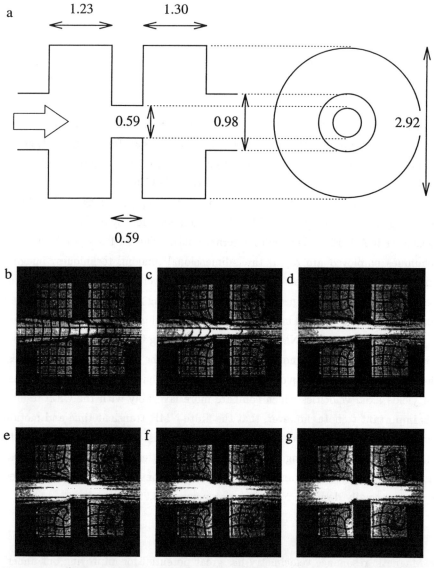

Figure 4:   a) Geometry of expansion-contraction-expansion-contraction pipe system (figures in cm). Arrow indicates the direction of fluid flow. In DANTE tagged velocimetry, a preparation sequence nulls sample magnetisation in orthogonal grid pattern (causing dark lines in the figure). The delay between this preparation and the imaging sequence is varied in each of a series of experiments. In (b) the delay is 90 ms. The fluid is water, flowing from left to right at 1.68 ml/s (mean velocity 6.77 cm/s in the central contraction). In each of (c) − (g) the delay is incremented by 180 ms.

Figure 5: Axial velocities in plane through centre of ECEC (Fig. 4). **a)** EPI velocimetry for 1.46 ml/s flow of 50 % by mass sucrose in tap water. Vertical axis shows $+x$ (cm/s) velocity. The x and y-axes are numbered in image pixels (0.07×0.07 cm). **b)**. EPI velocity map: bright represents $-x$ flow, dark $+x$. Velocities in central contraction corrupted by rapid motion during lengthy EPI transient (hence spike and blank pixels in **(a)** and **(b)**). **(c)** and **(d)** Gradient echo sequence (shorter transients) velocities for sucrose solution at 1.85 ml/s. **(e)** and **(f)** CFD velocities (FIDAP, Fluid Dynamics International) for flow at 1.85 ml/s.

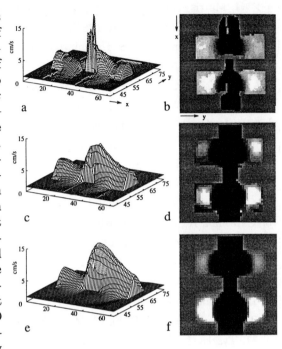

may prove useful for improved understanding of extensional flow effects in complex fluids and for validation of CFD models of processing equipment.

5. Acknowledgements

The authors acknowledge a benefaction from Dr. Herchel Smith that provided support and facilities and thank Dr. N. J. Herrod, Mr. J. A. Derbyshire, and Mr. D. Xing, for computer software and stimulating discussions.

6. References

[1] Lauterbur, P. C., Nature **242** 190-191 (1973).

[2] Mansfield, P. and P. K. Grannell, J. Phys. C **6** L422-426 (1973).

[3] P. Mansfield and P. K. Grannell, Phys. Rev. B **12** 3618-3634 (1975).

[4] M. K. Stehling, R. Turner, and P. Mansfield, Science **254**, 43-50 (1991).

[5] P. T. Callaghan Principles of Nuclear Magnetic Resonance Microscopy (Oxford University Press, 1991).

[6] P. G. Morris Nuclear Magnetic Resonance Imaging in Medicine and Biology (Clarendon Press, Oxford, 1986).

[7] W. A. Edelstein, J. M. S. Hutchinson, G. Johnson, and T. Redpath, Phys. Med. Biol. **25** 771 (1980).

[8] A. Haase, J. Frahm, D. Matthaei, W. Hanicke, and K.-D. Merbolt, J. Magn. Reson. **67** 258-265 (1986).

[9] L. D. Hall and T. A. Carpenter Magn. Reson. Imag. **10** 713-721 (1992).

[10] L. F. Gladden in Proceedings of ECAPT'94, ed. M. S. Beck *et al.* (UMIST, Manchester, 1994), pp. 466-477.

[11] Smith, M. A. Clin. Phys. Physiol. Meas. **11**, 101 (1990).

[12] Callaghan, P. T. and Y. Xia, J. Magn. Reson. **91** 326-352 (1991).

[13] Caprihan, A., and E. Fukushima, Physics Reports, **198** 195-235 (1990).

[14] G. Suryan, Proc. Indina Acad. Aci. **33** 107 (1951).

[15] E. O. Stejskal J. Chem. Phys. **43** 3597 (1965).

[16] G. A. Morris and R. Freeman J. Magn. Reson. **29** 433 (1978).

[17] L. Axel and L. Dougherty Radiology **171** 841-845 (1989).

[18] T. J. Mosher and M. B. Smith Magn. Reson. Med. **15** 334 (1990).

[19] M. Tyszka, N. J. Shah, R. C. Hawkes, and L. D. Hall Flow Meas. Instrum. **2** 127 (1991).

[20] K. Kose J. Magn. Reson. **98** 599-603 (1992).

[21] D. Xing, S. J. Gibbs, J. A. Derbyshire, E. J. Fordham, T. A. Carpenter, and L. D. Hall J. Magn. Reson. **106** 1-9 (1995).

[22] S. J. Gibbs, D. Xing, S. Ablett, I. D. Evans, W. Frith, D. E. Haycock, T. A. Carpernter, and L. D. Hall J. Rheol. **38** 1757-1767 (1994).

[23] Y. Xia, P. T. Callaghan and K. R. Jeffrey AIChE J. **38** 1408-1420, (1992).

[24] S. A. Altobelli, R. C. Givler, and E. Fukushima, J. Rheol. **35** 721-734 (1991).

[25] S. W. Sinton and A. W. Chow J. Rheol. **35** 735-772 (1991).

[26] C. J. Rofe, R. K. Lambert and P. T. Callaghan, J. Rheol. **38** 875-887 (1994).

[27] J. A. Derbyshire, S. J. Gibbs, T. A. Carpenter, and L. D. Hall AIChE J. **40** 1404-1407 (1994).

[28] J. M. Pope and S. Yao, Concepts in Magn. Reson. **5** 281-302 (1993).

[29] P. Boesiger, S. E. Maier, L. Kecheng, M. B. Scheidegger, D. Meier, J. Biomechanics, **25** 59-67 (1992).

Chapter 6

Microwave Tomography:
Optimization of the Operating Frequency Range

J.Ch.Bolomey
Supélec, Electromagnetics Department
Plateau de Moulon, 91190 Gif-sur-Yvette, France

1. Introduction

The microwave spectrum extends, more or less conventionally, from 300 MHz to 300 GHz. The wavelength (which is given by the formula $\lambda_0 = c/f$, where c=300,000 km/s is the light velocity in vacuum and f is the frequency) therefore lies between 1 m and 1 mm. This dimensional aspect is responsible for strong diffraction effects, which characterize microwave interactions with structures comparable in size to this wavelength domain. Furthermore, unlike other tomographic techniques based on X-rays, ultrasound, or nuclear magnetic resonance, these interactions are primarily dependent on the dielectric and magnetic constants of the materials under inspection. As a matter of fact, such constants are highly frequency-dependent for many materials. Consequently, it is not surprising that the selection of the operating frequency requires special attention in order to optimize the global performances of tomographic equipment. In most cases, the frequency is a "transparent" parameter. Indeed, the objective of the tomographic equipment is to retrieve a set of quantities of practical relevance for a given application. Such quantities may be of physical, chemical or physiological order: composition, faults, water content, temperature, and blood flow rate, are some illustrative examples. Microwaves only constitute one possible way to obtain these quantities and there is, *a priori* , a wide range of possible operating frequencies. However, there are some other particular (but important) cases where the choice of the operating frequency is imposed by users. These cases concern so-called microwave materials, that is to say materials to be used in the microwave frequency range, for applications such as anti-radar coatings or absorbers, transparent electromagnetic windows or radomes, and dielectric substrates for microwave circuit technology. In such applications, the quantity of practical relevance is directly related to the behavior of the material (absorption, transparency, dielectric and/or magnetic constants) in the frequency range where the material will be used. Consequently, the material inspection needs to be performed at these frequencies, and the frequency no longer constitutes a possible parameter to be adjusted in order to optimize the tomographic process performances. In this paper, attention is focused on the former situations where the frequency selection is open for optimization.

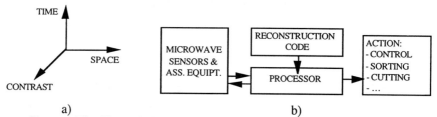

a)   b)

Figure 1: The 3D resolution space (a) and typical architecture of microwave equipment for on-line process tomography (b)

In practice, the possible usefulness of microwave tomographic techniques may extend over a wide range of applications with increasing complexity, from simple detection or localization to identification and absolute measurements. Despite a large variety of possible requirements, the global performances of tomographic equipment can be summarized in the 3D resolution space including spatial resolution, contrast and time resolution (Figure 1a). It can easily be presumed that the frequency has an evident and direct impact on all these three aspects. First of all, as shown later, spatial resolution is severely limited by diffraction phenomena to a fraction of the wavelength. Secondly, contrast is directly dependent on the sensitivity of the variations of the dielectric constant versus the quantity of practical relevance and such a sensitivity varies with frequency. Finally, time resolution is related to the number of data to be measured and processed, and this number is directly dependent on the dimension of the test object in terms of wavelength.

The block diagram of microwave process tomography equipment is very similar to any tomographic system, whatever its principle (Figure 1b). Typically, it can be considered as consisting of three main parts. The first part is formed by the sensors and the associated electronic or optoelectronic equipment to perform data acquisition. The second one performs the tomographic reconstruction process. The third part, finally, translates the results of the reconstructed data in quantities of practical relevance which can be used for control, sorting, or cutting purposes. If the impact of the operating frequency is evident on the first part of the equipment, its influence on the two following parts is less obvious. According to the selected reconstruction algorithm, it will be shown that it is possible to arrive at quite different conclusions.

Operational constraints impose the representative point to be located in some bounded domain of the 3D resolution space. If only one of the requirements cannot be fulfilled, for any reason, then the tomographic equipment will probably be useless for this application. It is known that there is, for a given equipment, some flexibility in moving in this 3D space to fit the requirements. For instance, contrast can be improved at the cost of degraded spatial and/or time resolutions, and conversely. Environmental considerations, operational contexts, electromagnetic compatibility requirements as well as cost aspects constitute key issues to be carefully analyzed in selecting the operating frequency range.

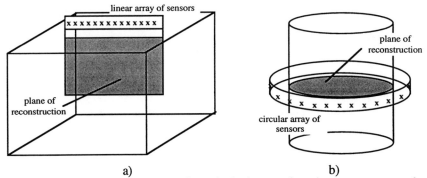

a)   b)

Figure 2: Two basic arrangements of practical relevance for microwave tomography:
(a) linear multi-frequency sensors for the detection of buried objects
(b) circular multi-incidence sensors for process tomography or biomedical imaging

After briefly reviewing the major characteristics of diffraction based interaction mechanisms with materials, the impact of frequency on different parts of the tomographic equipment will be discussed. Two arrangements of practical relevance in microwave tomography are considered. The first one consists of reflection probing or inspection of media accessible by only one side. This configuration is characteristic of applications aimed at the detection of buried objects in civil engineering, security or military contexts [25-28]. For these applications, probing can be performed from the analysis of the reflected field corresponding to multi-frequency interrogations. The second arrangement deals with cylindrical geometries. Such geometries can be used to model different applications relevant to process tomography in vessels [1,2] or to biomedical imaging [3-5]. In these configurations, the reconstruction process is often based on mono-frequency and multi-incidence transmission data.

2. Frequency Dependence of Dielectric Properties

The detection of inhomogeneities, such as small faults or defects, requires both 1) that the microwave interrogation beam penetrates the object under inspection and 2) that the defect has a sufficient effect on this beam to be effectively detected by a set of appropriate sensors. These two aspects are now successively considered under the frequency selection point of view. First of all, it is necessary that the attenuation constant remains reasonable at the operating frequency. In a homogeneous non-magnetic material, the complex propagation constant $\gamma=\alpha+j\beta$ is related to the complex dielectric constant $\varepsilon=\varepsilon'-j\varepsilon''=\varepsilon_0(\varepsilon'_r-j\varepsilon''_r)$ -- the index r refers to relative constants -- by

$$\gamma^2 = -\omega^2 \varepsilon \mu_0$$

where ε_0 and μ_0 designate the permittivity and the permeability of vacuum. The incident field distribution is well described as a function of the distance r by

$$E(r) = \frac{C\,e^{-\gamma r}}{r^v} = \frac{C\,e^{-\alpha r}\,e^{-j\beta r}}{r^v}$$

where C is a constant and $v=0$ for a quasi-plane wave collimated beam, $v=1/2$ for a cylindrical beam and $v=1$ for a spherical beam. The attenuation distance $L=1/\alpha$ is the distance over which the field is reduced by $1/e$ and is proportional to the transparency of the material. Consequently, the operating frequency must be chosen in such a way that the attenuation length L is not too small as compared to the required investigation depth through the material to be inspected. The space periodicity, which is fixed by the wavelength $\lambda = 2\pi/\beta$, will be shown to be closely related to the spatial resolution. Both L and λ can be deduced from ε and μ via the following formulas [6]:

$$\alpha = \frac{\pi\sqrt{2\varepsilon'_r}}{\lambda_0}\sqrt{\sqrt{1 + \tan\delta^2} - 1} \qquad \beta = \frac{\pi\sqrt{2\varepsilon'_r}}{\lambda_0}\sqrt{\sqrt{1 + \tan\delta^2} + 1}$$

where $\tan\delta = \varepsilon''_r / \varepsilon'_r$ is the loss factor. For low loss ($\tan\delta \ll 1$) and high loss ($\tan\delta \gg 1$) materials, these equations can be significantly simplified as follows:

$$\alpha = \frac{\pi\sqrt{\varepsilon'_r}\tan\delta}{\lambda_0} \qquad \beta = \frac{2\pi\sqrt{\varepsilon'_r}}{\lambda_0} \qquad (\tan\delta \ll 1)$$

$$\alpha = \beta = \sqrt{\pi\mu_0\sigma f} \qquad (\tan\delta \gg 1)$$

where $\sigma = \omega\varepsilon'\tan\delta$ is the equivalent conductivity of the material. Examples of low-loss materials are provided by standard plastics or ceramics, oil, alcohols, most gases, and dry or frozen media (soils, biological tissues, etc.), which exhibit loss ratios typically less than 10^{-2} up to 10 GHz. For such materials, the frequency dependence in the microwave frequency range is not very significant and can usually be neglected in the imaging process. On the contrary, high loss materials show non negligible frequency dependence. The manner the propagation constant γ is varying with frequency depends on the material.

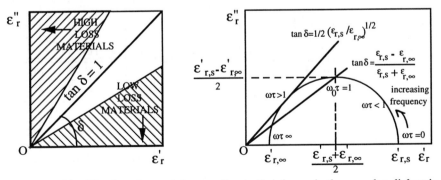

Figure 3: Classification of materials according to their losses in the complex dielectric permittivity plane (a) and the particular case of a Debye medium (b)

For instance, many liquids, and more particularly water, can conveniently be described by Debye models, or a combination of such models. According to this model, the real part ε'_r and the imaginary part ε''_r of the relative dielectric constant are given by the following formulas:

$$\varepsilon'_r = \varepsilon_{r,\infty} + \frac{\varepsilon_{r,s} - \varepsilon_{r,\infty}}{1 + (\omega\tau)^2} \qquad \varepsilon''_r = \frac{(\varepsilon_{r,s} - \varepsilon_{r,\infty})(\omega\tau)}{1 + (\omega\tau)^2}$$

with $\omega_0\tau = 1$ at the resonance frequency, $\varepsilon_{r,s}$ and $\varepsilon_{r,\infty}$ being the so-called static and optical permittivities. For pure water, the resonance frequency f_0 is close to 24 GHz at ordinary temperatures, with $\varepsilon_{r,s} \approx 80$ and $\varepsilon_{r,\infty} \approx 1$ around 25°C. This explains why microwaves are highly sensitive to water content of materials such as soils or biological tissues as shown on Table 1. On the contrary, for chilled water the resonance frequency f_0 drops down to 3 kHz at -10°C, with $\varepsilon_{r,s} \approx 95$ and $\varepsilon_{r,\infty} \approx 1$. Consequently, frozen soils or tissues are nearly transparent for microwaves. More generally, temperature has been shown to have a significant impact on the dielectric constant, especially on its imaginary part. For example, the temperature coefficient of soils [11] and biological tissues [12,13] is of the order of a few % per °C.

f GHz	λ_0 cm	\multicolumn{4}{c	}{MUSCLE (HWC)}	\multicolumn{4}{c	}{LUNG (MWC)}	\multicolumn{4}{c}{BONE (LWC)}
		ε'_r	σS/m	L cm	λ cm	ε'_r	σS/m	L cm	λ cm	ε'_r	σS/m	L cm	λ cm
0.433	69.3	53	1.43	3	8.5	36	0.72	4.7	10.8	5.6	0.08	16.3	28.2
0.915	33.8	51	1.60	2.5	4.4	35	0.73	4.5	5.4	5.6	0.10	12.8	13.7
2.450	12.3	49	2.21	1.7	1.8	32	1.32	2.3	2.2	5.5	0.16	7.9	5.2
5.800	5.2	43	4.73	0.8	0.8	28	4.07	0.7	1.0	5.1	0.26	4.7	2.3
10.000	3.0	40	10.3	0.3	0.5	25	9.08	0.3	0.6	4.5	0.44	2.5	1.4

f GHz	λ_0 cm	\multicolumn{4}{c	}{WET SOIL (HWC)}	\multicolumn{4}{c	}{MEDIUM SOIL (MWC)}	\multicolumn{4}{c}{DRY SOIL (LWC)}
		ε'_r	σS/m	L m	λ cm	ε'_r	σS/m	L m	λ cm	ε'_r	σS/m	L m	λ cm
0.100	300	26	.011	2.4	58.8	18	.0018	12.5	70.7	1.2	.0001	58	273
0.300	100	26	.037	0.73	19.6	18	.007	3.2	23.6	1.2	.0001	58	91.3
1.000	30	26	.2	0.13	5.86	18	.004	0.56	7.1	1.2	.00013	39	27.4
3.000	10	25	2.0	0.014	1.94	17	.5	0.044	2.4	1.2	.002	2.9	9.1
10.000	3	20	7.0	0.003	0.64	15	2.5	0.008	0.8	1.2	.04	.14	2.7

Table 1: Dielectric characteristics (ε'_r, σ), attenuation length (L) and wavelength (λ) of biological tissues [7,8] and soils [9,10] in the microwave frequency range, according to their water content (WC): low (LWC) ; medium (MWC) ; high (HWC)

3. Diffraction Based Interactions of Microwaves with Materials

For the tomographic detection of small local changes, a convenient test case is provided by a small spherical inclusion, located at point O (Figure 4) in a medium with propagation constant γ. Let a be the radius of the inclusion and ε_r its relative dielectric contrast with respect to the host medium. If illuminated by a locally plane wave, the inclusion behaves as a current element $\vec{I}$ which is related to the dielectric contrast and to

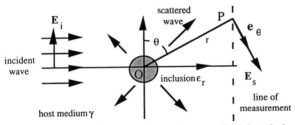

Figure 4: Scattering of a microwave beam by a small dielectric inclusion

the total field E_t by [14]

$$\vec{J} = j \, \omega \, \varepsilon \, [\, \varepsilon_r - 1] \vec{E}_t$$

This current is responsible for the scattered field $\vec{E_s}$ such that:

$$\vec{E}_s(r,\theta) = (\gamma a)^2 \, \frac{\varepsilon_r - 1}{\varepsilon_r + 2} \, \frac{a}{r} \, e^{-\gamma r} \, E_i(O) \sin \theta \, \vec{e}_\theta$$

This equation helps to explain the influence of the frequency. Firstly, for small inclusions with $|\gamma \, a| \ll 1$, the amplitude of the scattered field is proportional to $|\gamma a|^2$: the sensitivity of microwave imaging is then expected to be rapidly increased with the radius over wavelength ratio. Secondly, both the incident field at the inclusion location and the exponential propagation factor depend on the propagation constant γ in the host medium and, hence, may strongly depend on frequency as shown in the previous section. Furthermore, the explicit dependence with respect to ε_r demonstrates the non-linearity of the relationship existing between the scattered field and the dielectric contrast of the inclusion. With respect to possible changes of ε_r, the scattered field is the most sensitive for ε_r close to unity, that is to say for low contrast inclusions. For continuously changing materials, the total scattered field is related to the dielectric contrast distribution through an integral over the object [15]:

$$\vec{E}_S(\vec{r}) = [-\gamma^2 + \overrightarrow{\text{grad div}}] \int_{\text{OBJECT}} [\varepsilon_r(\mathbf{r}') - 1] \vec{E}_t(\vec{r}') \frac{e^{-\gamma|\vec{r}-\vec{r}'|}}{4\pi|\vec{r}-\vec{r}'|} d^3\vec{r}'$$

This integral can be considered as a superposition of the field scattered by small inclusions. It provides the mathematical basis for any microwave tomography reconstruction algorithm. In general, the tomographic process requires a non-linear inversion. However, under the assumption that the total field is known, for instance $\vec{E}_t \approx \vec{E}_i$ for low-contrast objects, the reconstruction can be linearized.

4. Tomographic Reconstruction Algorithms

The retrieval of the dielectric constant distribution from the measurement of the scattered field distribution depends on the measurement scheme and, more particularly, on the frequency. Figure 5a show the different ways of capturing scattered field data in the 3D measurement space. Both spectral (linear) and spatial (non-linear) techniques can be used.

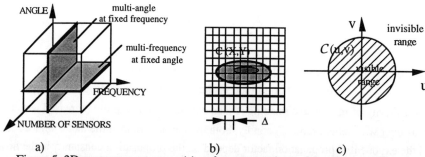

a)   b)   c)
Figure 5: 3D measurement space (a) and representations of the object under test: dielectric contrast C(X,Y) (b) and spectrum C(u,v) (c)

With spectral techniques, the object contrast C(X,Y) is retrieved from its 2D spectrum C(u,v) (Figure 5c) which is determined from 1D Fourier transforming the scattered field distribution corresponding to different projections. It is usually assumed that the scattered field has no evanescent wave contribution. In such a case, the spectrum can be determined only from the so-called visible range. As a result, the sampling rates of the projections are imposed by Shannon's sampling theorem: $\Delta x \leq \lambda/2$ for linear probing lines (Figure 6a) [17,18] and $\Delta\theta \leq \lambda/R_{min}$ for circular probing lines [16], R_{min} designating the radius of the minimum circle surrounding the object under test (Figure 6b). The spatial resolution mainly depends on the spectral plane filling. In transmission multi-incidence and mono-frequency tomography, each projection provides a circular arc of the object spectrum [17] (Figure 6c). By combining several projections, the spectrum can be determined in a circle of radius $\beta\sqrt{2}$, and the resulting

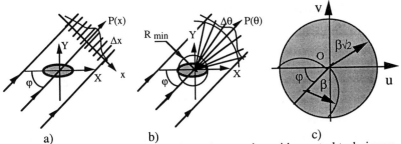

a)   b)   c)

Figure 6: Arrangements for microwave tomography with spectral techniques: Sampling rate for transmission/mono-frequency linear (a) and circular (b) probing, spectral plane filling from projections (c)

spatial resolution, defined as the width of the point space response, is around $\lambda/2$ whether the probing line is linear or circular. In reflection mono-incidence and multi-frequency tomography (Figure 7a), due to the non-uniform spectral plane filling (Figure 7b) [17,20], the spatial resolution depends on the direction: the transverse (or cross) spatial resolution ΔX and the longitudinal (or range) spatial resolution ΔY are given by [20,21]

$$\Delta X = .5\, \lambda_{min}/\tan\theta/2 \qquad\qquad \Delta Y \approx .5\, \lambda_{max}\lambda_{min}/(\lambda_{max}-\lambda_{min})$$

where θ is the angle under which the linear probe array is seen from a buried point, including possible refraction effects in case of non-contacting arrays (Figure 7a).

The range of usefulness of spectral techniques is limited to low contrast objects or to isolated targets. The linear reconstruction is efficiently real-time performed via Fast Fourier Transforms. Dealing with high contrast objects requires non-linear inversions.

With such spatial iterative techniques [e.g.22,23], the object is discretized according to a mesh size Δ, which is less than λ (Figure 5b).

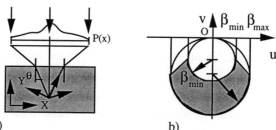

a)   b)

Figure 7: Arrangement for transmission multi-incidence/mono-frequency microwave tomography (a) and related filling of the spectral plane (b)

The discussion of the spatial resolution is not as easy as it is in the case of spectral techniques. From elementary considerations from information theory, the minimum number of linearly independent measurements must not be less than the number of unknowns. Practically, the effective spatial resolution seems to be less strictly limited by the wavelength and more dependent on the available signal over noise (s/n) ratio. Practically, successful reconstructions of moderately sized objects have been obtained with s/n ratios as low as 20 dB, with spatial resolutions of the order of $\lambda/5$ or $\lambda/20$, which are significantly better than the diffraction limit. Today, the major drawback of spatial iterative techniques results from the required computation effort. Existing codes are still incompatible with real time processing.

5. Design of the Tomographic Equipment

The design of the tomographic equipment requires a careful analysis of its expected functions. Basically, they consist 1) in producing an adequate set of illuminations of the object under test and 2) in measuring, for each illumination, the field scattered by this object. In multifrequency tomographic modalities, these two basic functions must be maintained within the whole operating frequency band. A first difficulty consists in producing a true plane or cylindrical wave, or at least a known incident field. The physical size of the antennas is usually of the order of the wavelength in the radiating medium. Their dimensions must accommodate the spatial illumination or sampling rate. However, at a fixed frequency, they could be significantly smaller at the cost of a reduced bandwidth and increased intercoupling. The incident field must be maintained, i.e. the antennas matched, whatever the object under test. Interactions between the sensors and the test object can be neglected for lossy materials. On the contrary, for low loss materials the coupling mechanisms must be integrated in the reconstruction process, at the cost of increased computation efforts. The effect of such a coupling is expected to increase when the frequency is decreased. The cost in designing and fabricating the sensor arrangement usually increases with frequency, except for some bands for public applications (satellite TV channels). MMIC (Monolithic Microwave Integrated Circuits) technologies offer rapid series arrangements of the sensors. However, they will become attractive only in case of large productions. More classical and cheaper multiplexed techniques, including the modulated scattering technique, have been investigated [24]. The selection of series or transmission arrangements of the sensors has to compromise time resolution and circuit complexity.

6. Conclusion

Microwaves are increasingly used as sensing agent for the tomographic inspection of opaque materials. The global performances of the tomographic process largely depends on the operating frequency or frequency band. Indeed, the selection of the operating frequency impacts both technological aspects related to the microwave part of the sensor and the data processing schemes which are required to achieve tomographic reconstructions. This paper has reviewed some of the key points to be addressed in the design of microwave tomographic equipment. The shape, dimensions and dielectric contrast of the material under inspection play a crucial role. Consequently, preliminary extensive dielectric characterization of small samples of materials must be performed. According to the transparency of the material, two distinct approaches can be considered. For low loss materials, the frequency must be increased as much as possible in order to increase spatial resolution via spectral techniques while maintaining sufficient sensitivity. This approach is particularly stimulated by the development of sources and circuits in the millimeter range corresponding to frequencies higher than 30 GHz. On the contrary, for lossy materials the frequency has to be decreased, possibly below 1 GHz, to provide acceptable s/n ratios. In these cases, spatial iterative techniques must be used to maintain the required spatial resolution. Non-negligible design problems are expected from interactions between sensors and test object at lower frequencies. These interactions can be taken into account in the reconstruction algorithm. In all cases, the immersion technique [29] of placing an external, or transition, medium with an appropriate dielectric constant between the sensors and the test object is efficient for at least three main reasons. Firstly, the spatial resolution is increased due to the fact that the wavelength is smaller than in air. Secondly, reflection losses are minimized and hence penetration is improved. Finally, external paths and possible interactions are significantly reduced.

To summarize, Table 2 shows some examples of microwave tomographic systems which have been recently developed, mainly for investigating buried objects in soils or concrete. Referring to the corresponding bibliography will illustrate how the operating frequency range has been selected, case by case, in order to obtain a good compromise between spatial resolution, penetration depth and operational flexibility.

Application	Ref	Sensors	Modality	Reconstruction Algorithm	Operating Frequency Range
Rebar detection in reinforced concrete	[25]	Linear, contacting 1T rans./32 Receiv.	Mono T Multi R Multi F	Spectral, linear Diffraction tomo.	7 GHz - 13 GHz swept frequency
Bridges and highways inspection	[21,26]	Linear, non contacting 1Trans./100 Receiv.	Mono T Multi R Multi F	Spectral, linear Diffraction tomo.	500 MHZ - 3.5 GHZ time domain
NDE and GPR	[27]	Linear, non contacting 5Trans./6 Receiv.	Multi T Multi R Multi F	Spatial, iterative non linear	2 GHz - 12 GHz swept frequency
Buried objects detection	[28]	Linear, non contacting 1Trans./32 Receiv.	Mono T Multi R Multi F	Spectral, linear Diffraction tomo.	400 MHz-1.2 GHz swept frequency time windowing

Table 2: Examples of microwave tomographic equipments
for the detection of buried objects

7. References

[1]   J. Ch. Bolomey, IEEE Trans. **MTT-37**:2109-2117 (1989).

[2]   N. Joachimowicz et al., in Proceedings of ECAPT '93, ed. M.S. Beck et al. (UMIST, Manchester, 1993) pp. 164-166.

[3]   L. E. Larsen and J. H. Jacobi, Diagn. Imag. Clin. Med. **11**:44-47 (1982).

[4]   J. C. Lin, Proc.IEEE **73**:374-375 (1985).

[5] J. Ch. Bolomey and M. S. Hawley, in Methods of Hyperthermia Control, M. Gautherie, ed. (Springer, Berlin, 1990) Section 2, pp. 35-111.

[6] A. R. Von Hippel, Dielectrics and Waves (Wiley, New York, 1954).

[7] E. C. Burdette et al., IEEE Trans. **MTT-28**:414-427 (1980).

[8] J. C. Lin, in Medical Applications of Microwave Imaging, L. E. Larsen and J. H. Jacobi, Editors, IEEE Pub. No. PC01941, pp. 13-40.

[9] J. E. Hipp, Proc.IEEE, **62**:98-103 (1974).

[10] M. T. Hallikainen et al., IEEE Trans. Geoscience and Remote Sensing **GE-23**:25-46 (1985).

[11] P. Hoekstra and A. Delaney, J. Geophysical Res. **79**:1699-1708 (1974).

[12] M. Miyakawa, Jap. J. Hyperthermic Oncology **4**:306-315 (1988).

[13] J. L. Guerquin-Kern et al., Bioelectromagnetics **6**:145-156 (1985).

[14] J. G. Van Bladel, Electromagnetic Fields (McGraw-Hill, New York, 1964).

[15] J. Ch. Bolomey and C. Pichot, Int. J. Imag Syst. and Tech. **2**:144-156 (1991).

[16] J. M. Rius et al., Electron Lett. **23**:564-565 (1987).

[17] M. Slaney et al., in Medical Applications of Microwave Imaging, L. E. Larsen and J. H. Jacobi, Editors, IEEE Pub. No. PC01941, pp. 184-212.

[18] C. Pichot et al., IEEE Trans. **AP-33**:416-425 (1985).

[19] J. M. Rius et al., IEEE Trans. Medical Imaging, **11**:233-246 and **11**:457-469 (1992).

[20] L. Chommeloux et al., IEEE Trans. **MTT-34**:1064-1076 (1986).

[21] E. J. Mast and E. M. Johanson, SPIE Proceedings Series **2275**, pp. 196-204.

[22] W. C. Chew and Y. M. Wang, IEEE Trans. Medical Imaging **9**:218:225 (1990).

[23] N. Joachimowicz et al., IEEE Trans. **AP-39**:1742-1752 (1991).

[24] J. Ch. Bolomey, SPIE Proceedings Series **2275**, pp. 2-10 (1994)

[25] C. Pichot and P. Trouillet, NATO Workshop on Bridges-ASCE Structures, A.S. Nowak, ed. (Kluwer Academic Publishers, Dordrecht 1991)

[26] J. P. Warhus et al., in SPIE Proceedings Series **2275**, pp. 178-185.

[27] W. H. Weedon et al., in SPIE Proceedings Series **2275**, pp. 156-167.

[28] Ph. Garreau et al., in Electromagnetic Environments and Consequences, Proceedings of Euroem'94, D. Sérafin et al. ed., 1664-1670.

[29] J. H. Jacobi et al., IEEE Trans. **MTT-27**:70-78 (1979).

Chapter 7

Optical Tomography

RC Darton, PD Thomas, PB Whalley
Department of Engineering Science,
University of Oxford, Parks Road, Oxford
OX1 3PJ.

1. Introduction

Many computerised tomography techniques have been developed for use in process engineering applications, mostly based on electrical signals (like capacitance), or on penetrating radiation (like X-rays). The use of visible light as the imaging radiation has, however, received very little attention, probably because the prime requirement has been to 'see' inside steel pipes or vessels, or into masses of solids, which are opaque. 'Optical' or 'visible light' tomography, does have several niche applications, of interest to process technologists, and deserves to be more widely known. We discuss here applications of optical tomography to gas jets, flames and to solid objects. At the present the three-dimensional information acquired is used for research purposes, but in the future it may also be found appropriate as providing input for process control.

1.1 Gas Jets

There are several methods described in the literature for measuring the 3-dimensional concentration field in a gas jet (Snyder and Hesselink[1]). These use elaborate optical arrangements, such as holographic interferometry, but do offer the possibility to record all necessary data in a very short time (less than a millisecond). A typical apparatus relies on a moving mirror to scan the beam across the test section. Fig.1 shows the result—in this case a concentration map for a helium jet in air, on a cross-section 6cm×6cm.

These methods measure optical path length, which with additional information about the system can be translated to gas density and composition. The methods can be extremely sensitive. Faris and Hertz[2] use a differential interferometer in which both interfering beams pass through the flow field, the two beams having differing polarizations. Fig.2 shows a reconstruction of an oxygen jet in air, the total error being estimated as better than 4.5% of the peak value. Faris and Byer[3] researching supersonic gas jets, have used a beam-deflection technique

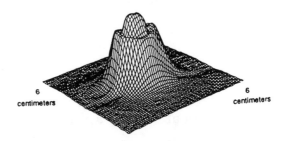

Figure 1: Helium concentration in a two dimensional slice through a jet flow
5.4 diameters downstream of the nozzle. Maximum value represents 100% pure
helium; the background is air (Snyder and Hesselink[4]).

which again measures optical path length, and hence gas density: this is precise
enough to measure the thickness of the shock front (around 80×10^{-6}m).

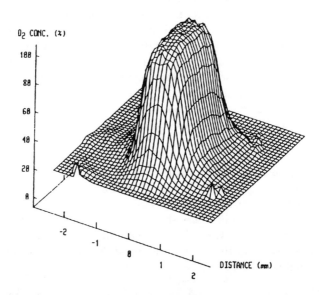

Figure 2: Tomographic reconstruction of the oxygen concentration in a rectangular
oxygen jet emerging into air (Faris and Hertz[2]).

1.2 Flames
Fischer and Burkhardt [5] use the visible radiation emitted by a flame to form an
image which is recorded by a video camera. A number of such images could be

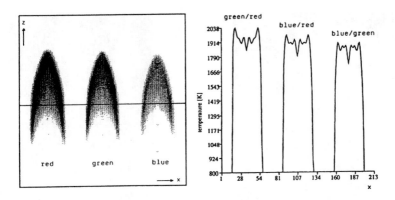

Figure 3: The left hand box shows three longitudinal sections through the reconstructed flame, each based on an image at a different wavelength. On the right are estimates of the flame temperature, derived from pairs of the red, green and blue reconstructions.

used to reconstruct the three-dimensional model, though in this case the authors assumed cylindrical symmetry, which enables reconstruction from a single image. This *emission* tomography is the inverse of *absorption* tomography, since the intensity of the image *increases* with the path length through the object (flame). Fischer and Burkhardt used a colour camera with lens and filters recording three distinct images at different wavelengths, from which a temperature map could be constructed (fig.3). Burkhardt [6] showed how such images could be used to control the combustion process.

1.3 Solid Objects
Kawata *et al.* [7] have described an optical microscope technique in which the set

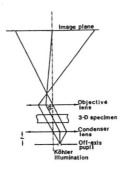

Figure 4: Optical microscope arrangement

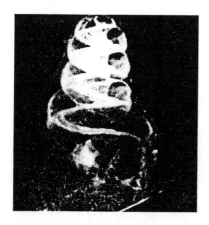 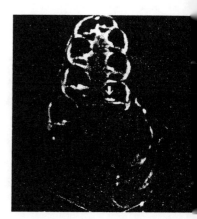

Figure 5: Tomographic reconstruction, using visible light, of the inner ear of a guinea pig; left, one projection, right, a cross-section through the tomographic model (Brown *et al.* [10]).

of images is generated by a microscope with an off-axis pupil rotating about the axis of the microscope objective (fig.4). The limited angle of view does lead to difficulties in reconstruction, and ultimately to loss of resolution. The authors used the technique to determine the structure of the single-celled Spirogyra organism. This technique has been developed further [8,9].

An optical tomography system for looking at the structure of 'thick objects' was described by Brown *et al.* [10]. The object is rotated in the immersion chamber, illuminated by a beam of filtered light from a tungsten source. Fluid in the immersion chamber reduces the effect of refraction at the object's surfaces. Fig.5 shows an example reconstruction—the decalcified inner ear (cochlea) of a guinea pig—based on a set of 96 projections, evenly spaced over 180 degrees. Light absorption is measured, so the object must be translucent.

2. Optical Tomography of Foams

Foaming occurs in equipment for distillation and absorption, boiling heat transfer, in aerated fermenters and process piping. Characterising the structure of a foam, *in situ*, can be important for various reasons. Predicting how much unwanted foam is present in a process vessel involves not just knowledge of the surface properties, but also of the drainage - which depends on the foam structure. The rates of mass transfer between gas and liquid will depend on interfacial area, and transfer coefficients in lamella and Plateau border. (The Plateau borders are the prism-shaped edges where three lamellae meet). With solid foams, flexible or rigid, the mechanical properties depend crucially on the structure.

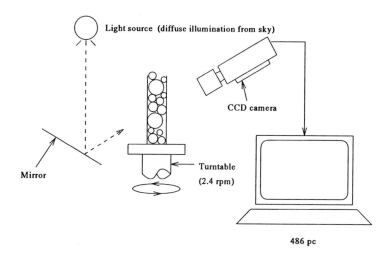

Figure 6: Apparatus for visible light tomography of foam.

Rhodes and Khaykin[11] have used stereology, determining average volume properties from a two-dimensional foam cross-section. For a solid foam, the two-dimensional cross-section can be obtained by casting the foam in resin or wax, and cutting slices. This is a lengthy process, and anyway clearly unsuitable for gas/liquid foams. Morris and Morris[12] used X-ray computerised tomography to resolve a two-dimensional cross section of a liquid foam in a beaker. The need to measure foam structure has led to our interest in tomography.

2.1 Development of an Imaging System

Our vision system has much in common with the early types of X-ray CT machines, where a solid model is constructed from information given by the attenuation of many rays though an object[13], and is similar in concept to the system used by Brown *et al.* [10]. Diffuse light is used to illuminate the foam in order to prevent specular reflections. Light scattered by the Plateau borders in the foam gives rise to shadows on the image formed at the camera lens. A video system is used to sample a large number of images from a 360° arc around a foam sample, and a voxel representation of the Plateau border geometry is constructed.

The use of visible light in this way has several advantages over the use of X-rays, and one major drawback. Apart from the ease of use and relatively lower cost of an electronic camera compared with X-ray sources and detectors, the visible light system does not suffer from beam hardening, the image-distorting effect caused when multi-frequency X- rays are attenuated according to wavelength, rather than uniformly across the band. It is difficult to produce monochromatic X-radiation, so this problem always exists to some extent. With visible light and aqueous foams, light is scattered much more uniformly over the spectrum.

The disadvantage with using visible light attenuation for a tomography experiment with a non-translucent object is that it is only possible to create a binary Radon transform (see below), resulting in a loss of information per image. Because the Plateau borders scatter light almost completely, it is not possible to tell if an individual light ray has passed through more than one Plateau border. This can lead to difficulties in the reconstruction if there are parts of the structure where many Plateau borders are close to each other, though the excellent spatial resolution of the images tends to compensate this.

Our experimental arrangement is shown in fig.6. The sample is placed on a turntable which rotates at a fixed slow rate. This enables the foam to be photographed from a 360 degree arc. The illumination is provided by reflecting an image of the sky outside the laboratory window off a mirror behind the foam which gives a good diffuse light illumination and prevents specular reflections in liquid foams.

The Dage-MTI 72S CCD camera gives a PAL output signal from a matrix of 750×580 active elements, which is fed into a 486PC running Video for Windows with a VideoLogic Captivator card. The video system can cope with varying frame sizes and frame rates, but is constrained by the bandwidth of the PC backplane, which seems to be about 500kB per second with Video for Windows running. The system can sample 24 frames per second at a resolution of 160×120 pixels. The 8-bit voxel models are thresholded to produce binary voxel sets. There is no obvious automatic thresholding procedure, so the threshold is selected by hand for each reconstruction to optimise the clarity of the final image.

It is important to check the correct alignment of the camera before taking a video clip. The axis of the camera must be aligned at a known angle to the axis of rotation of the turntable, though the axis of rotation does not have to be exactly in the centre of the image. When the images are cropped later, a small discrepancy in the positioning of the centre of rotation can be easily corrected. Also, the camera is initially focussed on the foam with no background illumination and at as large an aperture as possible. This gives the smallest depth of field, and it is possible to set the focus to be at the centre of the foam. When background illumination is used and the lens aperture stopped down, the depth of field will expand so that the whole foam sample will be in focus. Typically the sample space will be around 1cm^3 with the lenses now used.

When using aqueous foams, they must be stable and not change configuration for the duration of the video capture. In one revolution of the turntable, the system could capture 600 frames at the specified resolution, but the results we present here have been reconstructed from 140 frames. In an optimal CT system,

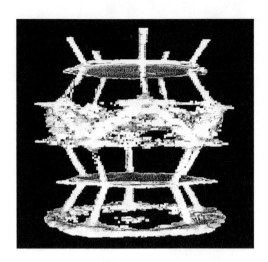

Figure 7: A tomographic reconstruction of a dodecahedral bubble in which the axis of rotation is orthogonal to the axis of the camera lens[14].

the voxel dimension, number of frames and image dimension are about the same. In this case, sampling many more than 140 frames does not add to image quality.

In our initial work, Thomas et al. [14], the axis of the camera lens was orthogonal to the (vertical) axis of rotation of the foam. This configuration had one major disadvantage. Adjacent Plateau borders in the horizontal plane were reconstructed as a disk, since, during rotation the borders obstruct each other and information is lost (fig.7). This problem can be solved by putting the camera at an angle to the axis of rotation, as shown in fig.6—we currently use 60°. Clearly there is an optimum angle, because moving the angle of the camera until it is on the axis of rotation again loses information, because every image will then be congruent.

2.2 Working with Solid Foams
These do not need to be contained in a glass vessel, and do of course maintain a stable shape for as long as it takes to gather the image data. Fig.8 shows one frame from a series of images of a polyurethane foam sample, and the quality of such pictures is such that no retouching is necessary. Fig.9 shows a single view of the tomographic reconstruction.

2.3 Working with Liquid Foams
When dealing with gas/liquid foams, which are composed of lamellae and Plateau borders, the pictures from the camera are not directly suitable for use in a CT reconstruction algorithm. Any shadows caused by cell facets at an angle nearly

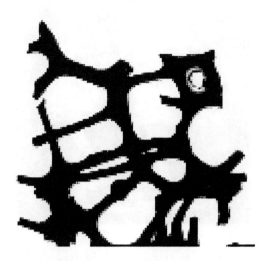

Figure 8: Single video image of a polyurethane foam sample.

parallel with the axis of the lens will disrupt the reconstruction process. These polygonal shadows are best removed with a line detector program which can enhance lines in an image (the Plateau borders) and remove areas of continuous shadow. The algorithm for this operation is simply a set of 7×7 pixel convolutions which match lines at various angles in an image[15]. An example of the process is shown in figs.10a and 10b. Fig.10a is the unretouched video signal from the camera, and fig.10b is the result of the edge-enhancing process.

The algorithm used to build a computational model of the foam is simple back projection. For every image, rays are traced through each voxel and through the image to the centre of the camera lens, as simulated by the computer. The value of a voxel is increased depending on the intensity of the pixel in the image through which the ray is being traced. At the end of this operation, the values are normalised to lie on the interval 0..255 so that each voxel is represented by a single byte.

Our best results come from experiments on dryish foams. Liquid foams stabilised by detergent are typically stable for tens of minutes and after about 30 minutes the Plateau borders are easy to photograph. Using a tube of 12mm diameter, it is possible to produce foams with three bubble-widths across. This allows us to photograph the middle bubbles without incurring the refractive distortion at the edges of the tube.

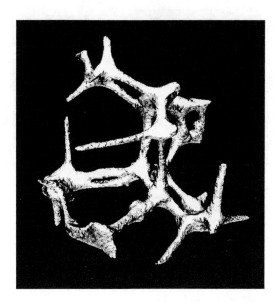

Figure 9: Tomographic reconstruction of the polyurethane foam sample.

Fig.11 shows a voxel model of a 14-sided bubble, having two hexagonal and twelve similar pentagonal sides. The individual bubbles are of the order of 4mm across.

3. The Potential of Optical Tomography

Optical tomography using interferometry is a sensitive technique for detecting spatial variation in a gas mixture, suitable for use in a laboratory environment. Visible light emission tomography has proved to be a useful method for measuring the temperature gradients in flames. Detecting emissions at different wavelengths also opens the possibility of determining the local composition of the flame, through the emission spectra.

The improving performance of CCD cameras and computer equipment, means that faster image capture rates, perhaps using multiple cameras, are becoming more feasible. This will increase the number of areas in which optical tomography can be applied.

As yet little has been done with colour photography. Using coloured tracers to visualise flow patterns in vessels is a possibility, as is the use of liquid crystals to indicate local temperature variations. This is in addition to the use of emission spectra.

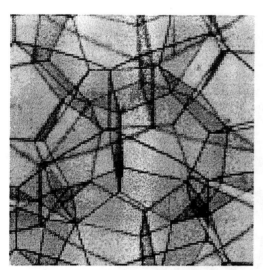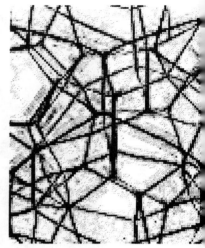

Figure 10: Left (a), unretouched video image of air/water foam; right (b) edge-enhanced video image of air/water foam.

On the processing side, there is a need to increase the speed and efficiency of the reconstruction software. The simple algorithm we used is $O(mn^3)$, where m is the number of images used and n is the dimension of the voxel set. Since n must increase as the video bandwidth increases to maintain optimal reconstruction, the problem quickly becomes much more complex with increasing data size. Suppose we wanted to use 500 frames of 500×500 pixels resolution and reconstruct to give a 500×500×500 voxel model, the video bandwidth required would be about 5MB per second and the storage required to contain the volume model would be 125MB. In our case, increased model resolution would mean that clusters of bubbles could be studied and average properties measured, which seems important for foam characterisation.

The advantages of being able to use readily available video and image processing equipment are considerable: ease of use, speed, and safety. The disadvantage is that it is only possible to deal with objects whose details can be 'seen'. At present this restricts analysis to samples which are translucent, or to structures which contain at most a few percent solid or liquid matter.

4. Conclusions

Optical tomography has been developed, principally using interferometry, to examine composition fields in gas flows. This is a technique of considerable potential interest to chemical engineers interested in turbulence and mixing, re-

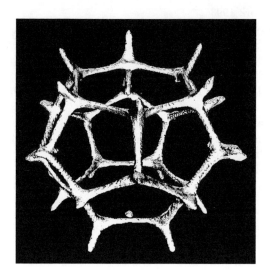

Figure 11: Voxel model of 14-sided bubble in air/water foam stabilised with Teepol.

acting flows and visualisation of flow fields.

It is possible to perform computerised tomography experiments on solid objects using visible light instead of gamma or X-rays, a good method for semi-transparent materials or open structures. Suitable optical or processing equipment is becoming cheaper and more readily accessible. Future opportunities include the use of wavelength information (colour) in tracing flow patterns or temperature variations in processing equipment.

Acknowledgements

Financial support by Shell Research BV is gratefully acknowledged. Thanks also to Theo Platt for supplying figs. 9 and 11.

References

[1] R Snyder and L Hesselink, Appl. Opt. **24** 4046–4051 (1985)
[2] GW Faris and HM Hertz, Appl. Opt. **28** 4662–4667 (1989)
[3] GW Faris and RL Byer, Appl. Opt. **27** 5202–5212 (1988)
[4] R Snyder and L Hesselink, Opt. Lett. **13** 87–89 (1988)
[5] W Fischer and H Burkhardt, SPIE **1349** 96–105 (1990)
[6] H Burkhardt, in Proceedings of the International Seminar on imaging in transport processes, eds. S Sideman and K Hijikata (Athens May 1992) Publ. Begell

House Inc, New York 1993

[7] S Kawata, O Nakamura and S Minami, J. Opt. Soc. Am. A **4** 292–297 (1987)

[8] O Nakamura, S Kawata and S Minami, J. Opt. Soc. Am. A **5** 554–561 (1988)

[9] S Kawata, O Nakamura, T Noda, H Ooki, K Ogino, Y Kuroiwa and S Minami, Appl. Opt. **29** 3805–3809 (1990)

[10] CS Brown, DH Burns, FA Spelman, AC Nelson, Appl. Opt. **31** 6247–6254 (1992)

[11] MB Rhodes and B Khaykin, Langmuir 643–649 (1986)

[12] RM Morris and A Morris, Chem. and Ind. 1902–1903 (1965)

[13] H Scudder, Proc. IEEE **24** 628–637 (1978)

[14] PD Thomas, RC Darton and PB Whalley, Chem. Eng. J. **56** 187–192 1995

[15] J Canny, IEEE Trans. on Pat. Anal. Mach. Int. **PAMI-8** 679–697 (1986)

Chapter 8

Principles of Mutual Inductance Tomography

A J Peyton
Dept. of Electrical Engineering and Electronics
University of Manchester Institute of Science and Technology
Manchester M60 1QD U.K.

A R Borges
Départmento de Electrónica e Telecomunicações
Universidade de Aveiro
Aveiro 3800 Portugal

1. Introduction

1.1 Background

A wide variety of tomography techniques have been researched or considered for process applications as is evident from the content of many of the chapters contained in this book. Electrical techniques in particular, despite their relatively modest image resolution, have received much attention recently, mainly because of their potentially high imaging speeds, relatively low cost, non-intrusive and non-hazardous nature. The combination of these properties makes electrical techniques attractive for a number of process applications especially on-line monitoring and control.

Electrical techniques can themselves be further sub-divided and considerable interest has been given to the methods based on the measurement of the passive electrical quantities, namely resistance (impedance), capacitance and inductance. Electrical Impedance Tomography (EIT) is based on the measurement of resistance and reactance patterns [1,2] and can produce conductivity (σ) and permittivity (ε) images. Electrical Capacitance Tomography (ECT) involves the measurement of capacitance profiles [3,4] and generates images of permittivity distributions. Mutual inductance tomography, or Electromagnetic Inductance Tomography (EMT), as it is sometimes termed, completes the set of these techniques and at present is the least well developed. EMT employs inductance measurements to extract tomographic data related to permeability (μ) and conductivity distributions and is the subject of this chapter.

1.2   Overview of the Technique

An overview of a typical EMT system is present in Fig. 1, and consists of the usual three main sub-systems: the sensor array, the control electronics and the host computer.

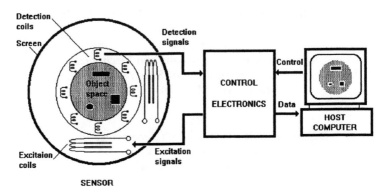

Fig. 1   Block diagram of a typical mutual tomography system.

The sensor array operates in the usual manner associated with tomographic systems. The object space is energised by a sinusoidally varying AC magnetic field created by one or more of the excitation coils. This creates a projection which can interrogate the object material. A number of projections are taken in sequence as dictated by the control electronics and for each projection, the peripheral field values are measured with the detection coils. It is the use of coils as detection magnetometers which lead to the term mutual inductance tomography since it is the mutual coupling between the excitation coils and the detection coils which is being measured. Naturally other types of magnetometer could be used. The measured signals are subsequently digitised and fed to the host computer which operates an image reconstruction algorithm in order to create an image or extract some other tomographic data, for example a component fraction.

1.3   Other Similar Techniques

In addition to EMT there are a number of related electrical techniques, which employ AC magnetic excitation. For example, EIT systems have been demonstrated in which the object space is magnetically excited with a set of induction coils. In these systems, the flow of excitation current is induced rather than being injected directly through the electrodes [5]. Another example is the combination of tomographic techniques to conventional induction flowmeters [6,7], which is a recent advance on the well established Faraday effect used for measuring flow in conductive liquids. Multiple electrodes are being combined with a rotating parallel magnetic excitation field to create the tomographic sensor.

2.   Physical Principle

A considerable amount of work has been reported on the solution of field equations for different electromagnetic applications involving inductance. Examples closely related to EMT are by Moran and Kunz [8] for oil well logging and Harpen [9] for NMR applications. A formal description of a measuring system based on electromagnetic inductance can begin with Maxwell's equations, given in complex vector notation as:

$$\underline{\nabla} \times \underline{E} = -j\omega \underline{B} \quad (1) \qquad\qquad \underline{\nabla} \times \underline{H} = (\sigma + j\omega\epsilon)\underline{E} \quad (2)$$

$$\underline{\nabla} \cdot \underline{D} = q \quad (3) \qquad\qquad \underline{\nabla} \cdot \underline{B} = 0 \quad (4)$$

If we assume that the object material has linear and isotropic electrical and magnetic properties then,

$$\underline{B} = \mu\underline{H} \quad (5) \qquad\qquad \underline{D} = \epsilon\underline{E} \quad (6) \qquad \underline{J} = \sigma\underline{E} \quad (7)$$

For the practical case, we can make a number of simplifications such as, (i) assume the two dimensional case (x,y plane), (ii) ignore the effects of displacement current which may be negligible for the frequencies and materials of interest here (ie. $j\omega\epsilon \ll \sigma$), and (iii) neglect free charges ($q = 0$, which follows from i and ii previously). Then combining equations we have,

$$\underline{\nabla} \times [\sigma(x,y)^{-1}[\underline{\nabla} \times (\mu(x,y)^{-1}\underline{B}(x,y))]] = -j\omega\underline{B}(x,y) \quad (8)$$

and
$$\underline{\nabla} \cdot \underline{B}(x,y) = 0 \quad (9)$$

The tomographic problem is therefore to excite the object space with a number of field strength patterns and then measure the field components for each pattern around the outside of the space. A sufficient number of excitation patterns and field measurements must be used to enable an image of adequate quality to be reconstructed and accurate image reconstruction would require a complex non-linear or iterative reconstruction algorithm to take into account the double curl nature in the actual field distributions. In addition, to gain the maximum amount of information from the object space, the real and imaginary parts of both the radial and tangential vector field components should be measured. For simplicity, however, most practical systems ignore the tangential components and only recently has phase information been considered.

To proceed further, it is convenient to introduce the magnetic vector potential $\underline{A}$ and electric scalar potential Φ with properties,

$$\underline{H} = \nabla \times \underline{A} \quad (10) \qquad\qquad \underline{E} = -j\omega\mu\underline{A} - \nabla\Phi \quad (11)$$

Combining eq.'s (2), (10) and (11) and using a well known vector identify, we have for each region in the object space,

$$\nabla^2 \underline{A} = j\omega\mu\sigma\underline{A} \qquad (12)$$

If we consider a simple example of a circular target object in the centre of a circular unscreened object space as shown in Fig. 2, then expressions for the magnetic field can be obtained by integrating eq. (12) over both the target and air regions and incorporating suitable boundary conditions [10].

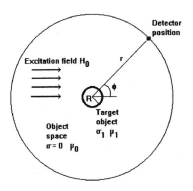

Fig. 2   Simple example of a circular target object in a traverse parallel field.

The radial magnetic field H_R at the detector position (r, ϕ) in circular coordinates is given [10] below, where $k^2 = \omega\mu\sigma$ and H_0 is the applied excitation field assumed to be parallel.

$$H_R = H_0 . \cos\phi . [1 + \frac{R^2}{r^2} G(kR)] \qquad (13)$$

The function G is defined in terms of Bessel functions of the first kind of order 0 and 2, as given by their subscripts.

$$G(kR) = \frac{(\mu_1 - \mu_0).J_0(j^{\frac{3}{2}}kR) + (\mu_1 + \mu_0).J_2(j^{\frac{3}{2}}kR)}{(\mu_1 + \mu_0).J_0(j^{\frac{3}{2}}kR) + (\mu_1 - \mu_0).J_2(j^{\frac{3}{2}}kR)} \qquad (14)$$

Fig. 3 shows a plot of the real and imaginary parts of G as a function of the dimensionless quantity kR. The function G can be considered as a "shape factor" which takes into account the tendency of the magnetic field to distort around the target object. The "shape factor" contains both real and imaginary parts and as can be seen the real part decreases monotonically from 0 to -1, while the imaginary part has a distinct minimum value.   Note that for a given radius, permeability and conductivity there exists an optimum frequency which gives the maximum change in the imaginary component.   This could be exploited in an EMT system to yield maximum sensitivity to a component of interest and possibility to perform spectroscopy (to obtain selective sensitivity to objects by varying the frequency). From a practical point of view, this optimum frequency can only be obtained for moderately conducting materials. Another important point to note from eq. (14) is that the shape factor G is dependant on the term $kR = R.(\omega\sigma\mu)$. Clearly, to image low conductivity materials requires a high excitation frequency.

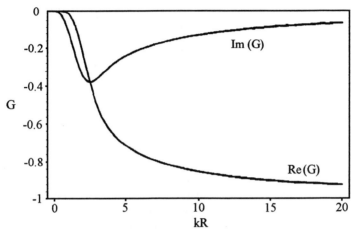

Fig. 3   The real and imaginary parts of G as a function of kR.

3.   Overview of Some Existing Systems

Three different examples of EMT systems are described in this section. These examples reflect the variety of possible configurations. The three systems also employ different operating frequencies for detecting different types of object material.

3.1   An experimental biomedical system

Fig. 4 shows a simplified diagram of a two coil experimental biomedical system [11]. The object to be imaged is situated on a turntable which can be drawn in a horizontal plane along the line of symmetry between the two coils. Coil C_1 is used for excitation purposes and is a 160 turn solenoid. Coil C_2 is also a solenoid but with 80 turns. Both coils are covered with a grounded electrostatic screen to ensure the coupling mechanism between the coils is predominantly inductive as opposed to capacitive. The excitation coil is driven from a sinusoidal supply at 2 MHz and the detection coil forms a resonant circuit with the capacitance of the connecting cables and detection circuitry which is tuned to the excitation frequency. The object was scanned between the coils at typically a few cm per second to produce each projection and the turntable could be rotated to obtain as many projections as required. The recorded data was fed into an image reconstruction computer and images were reconstructed using both back projection and filtered back projection algorithms, as described in section 4.

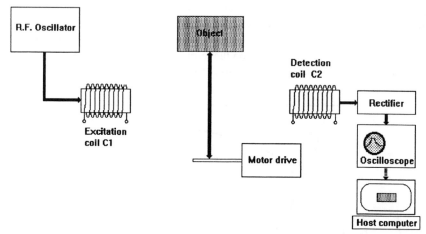

Fig. 4   Schematic diagram of an experimental two coil tomographic system

The system was used to image a variety of phantom objects such as a circular (diameter 10.2 cm) beaker and a square (side 22.5 cm) and a rectangular (sides 14 cm by 10.5 cm) plastic tank each filled with saline (concentration 0.1 mole/l). In addition, aluminium cylinders were also placed inside the tanks in some applications in order to assess the potential of the technique for determining the shape of internal features. In general, a relatively small number of projections, typically up to 12, was used for reconstruction.

3.2   A multiple pole system

Fig. 5 shows a block diagram of a multiple pole EMT system developed at the University of Aveiro. The system employs a lower excitation frequency to that in Fig. 4 and consequently can only detect higher conductivity materials. Other notable differences are that the system has an external magnetic shield which concentrates the field inside the object space to increase sensitivity and which also minimises external interference. In addition, the use of multiple excitation/detection coils avoids the need for mechanical scanning.

The sensor has a similar structure to some ECT systems, but with the electrode plates being exchanged for excitation/detection coils. There are 16 such coils and each coil consists of small winding on a ferrite core. The object space has a diameter of 150 mm and is surrounded by a magnetic confinement shield, with an axial length of 100 mm, constructed from compressed ferrite powder. Each coil together with its associated electronics can perform either excitation or detection functions as directed by the host computer and at any moment in time one coil is energised in order to create a projection whilst the remaining 15 coils act as detectors. Each coil is energised in sequence to give a total of 16 projections and for each projection, both the magnitude and phase (with respect to the excitation waveform) of the signals from the remaining 15 coils is measured. Therefore a total of 16x15x2 = 480 measurements are available per frame. Some initial results associated with this system are shown later in section 4.

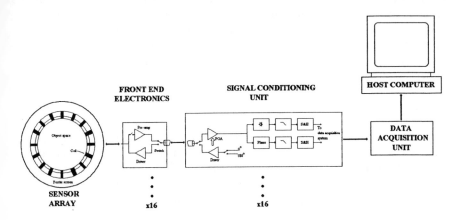

Fig. 5   Block diagram of a multiple pole EMT system at the University of Aveiro.

3.3   *A parallel excitation field system*

Figure 6 shows an overview of an inductive EMT system which employs a parallel excitation field [12] when the object space is empty. The use of a parallel excitation field is intended to maximise the relative sensitivity at the centre of the object space with respect to the edges.

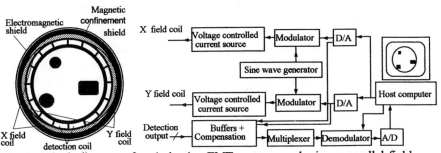

Fig. 6   Block diagram of an inductive EMT system employing a parallel field

The primary sensor in this system has an internal diameter of 75 mm and is composed of four assemblies, namely, excitation coils, detection coils, a magnetic confinement screen and an external conducting screen. The excitation coil consists of two pairs of orthogonal (X and Y) windings. Each winding surrounds the object space and has an appropriate turns density to ensure that a parallel uniform magnetic field is created within the object space when it is empty [18].   The applied field has a frequency of

500 kHz and the direction of the field can be controlled over 360^0 by the relative magnitudes of the excitation currents in the X and Y windings. The currents are controlled by the image reconstruction computer and a large number of field projections are possible. There are 21 individual detection coils, which are equally positioned round the circumference, enabling 21 concurrent measurements of the peripheral field to be acquired for each particular field projection. The ferrite magnetic confinement shield both concentrates the field inside the space to increase sensitivity and prevents interference from external objects. The conducting shield further confines the flux and improves electromagnetic compatibility.

4.   Reconstruction Methods

A number of different reconstruction techniques have been applied to EMT systems described in the previous section. The reconstruction algorithms include simple heuristic methods, linear back projection and filtered linear back projection, weighted linear back projection and arithmetic reconstruction techniques. These different approaches are described in the following sub-sections.

4.1   *Heuristic image reconstruction*

Simple image reconstruction algorithms can be devised for EMT systems in certain situations by assuming a priori knowledge of the object being imaged. These types of algorithms require a very simplified problem, for example locating the position of a single target object of known geometry and material in an object space which is otherwise non-magnetic and non conductive. Experiments at the University of Aveiro on this approach have shown that it is possible to determine the (x,y) position and diameter of a target of circular cross-section with good results using the multi-pole system described in section 3.2. Simple empirical formulae are used to extract this information from the sensor measurements.

Clearly this approach can only be applied to a very limited number of situations, however the approach is simple and the algorithms run virtually in real time on even relatively low powered host computers. The approach may be suitable for tracking the position of a magnetically labelled target particle or locating the position of a metallic tool tip.

4.2   *Linear and filtered linear back projection*

When an object was scanned between the detection and excitation coils of the two coil system described in section 3.1, the signal from the detection coils changed significantly as the object passed through the line connecting the two coils. The signal response was similar to a hard field system and consequently it was reasonable to test conventional hard field reconstruction algorithms on this system. The images produced, as shown in Fig. 7, were clearly representative of the actual objects and very encouraging. The figures shows an image of the same box also obtained by filtered back projection from 12 projections, with two aluminium cylinders placed inside the tank This time the image is represented in a contour map format and the outlines of the two cylinders can be seen inside the tank as well as the outline of the tank.

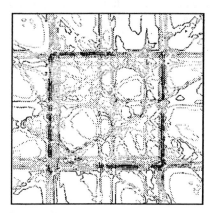

Fig. 7   Typical image obtained from the two coils system described in section 3.1
(Courtesy Al-Zeibak and Saunders University of Wales, Swansea)

The system clearly demonstrates the potential of the inductive approach for imaging conducting aqueous solutions with electromagnetic properties typical of those found in biomedical applications.

4.3   Weighted linear back projection

Weighted linear back projection using sensitivity maps is a widely used method of image reconstruction for electrical tomographic systems and has also been applied to EMT. As an example, the image reconstruction algorithm described here was used with the parallel field system described earlier in section 3.3. The algorithm was derived as follows. Firstly the forward problem was solved by an experimental method of inserting a copper test bar in turn into every pixel location inside the object space. This provided the forward response of the system to every pixel. These data were then organised into a transformation matrix to convert all the sensor measurements into an image. The forward problem can also be solved using finite element electromagnetic simulation or by direct analytical means.

Fig. 8 shows the images of several conductivity distributions obtained using these 5 field projections. Fig 8(a) shows a single 15 mm diameter copper tube (left) together with a three dimensional graphic representation (right) of the same image. This image was obtained using 5 equally spaced field projections with angles of 0^0, 72^0, 144^0, 216^0 and 288^0.

Fig. 8(b) shows two copper rods, Fig. 8(c) shows a single coper rod in the centre and

Fig. 8(d) shows a half filled object space with aluminium foil. Clearly the images show the correct characteristics of the actual contents of the object space. Similar images were obtained from this system when ferrite rods were inserted into the object space. Conductive material tends to exclude flux and produces positive pixel values, whereas ferrite material tends to concentrate flux and produce negative pixel values. Although these images were obtained using solid targets, equivalent images would be obtained with similar target distributions of conductive or ferromagnetic particles such as metal filing or crushed, fired ferrite powder.

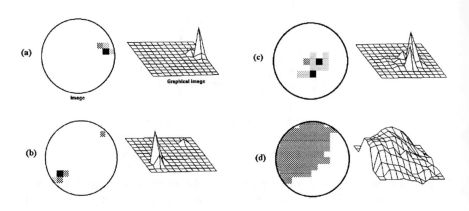

Fig. 8   Reconstructed images from the parallel field system.
(a) Single 15 mm copper bar positioned top left.   (b) Two copper bars
(c) Copper bar in the centre.   (d) Half filled object space with aluminium foil.

Of course the images from this system are poor since they are based on a small number of projections and consequently only 5 x 21= 105 measurements are available for reconstruction. In addition, no attempt has been made to increase artificially the apparent resolution by adding a greater number of pixels than data. Naturally, the image quality would be expected to improve significantly if more projections were used. Consequently image fidelity is poor especially in the central region as shown in Figure 8(c).

4.4   *Arithmetic reconstruction techniques (ART)*

ART has recently been applied to simulated data from the Aveiro multiple pole system, with promising results as shown in the following diagram with a 10 mm ferrite cylinder placed 36 mm from the centre.

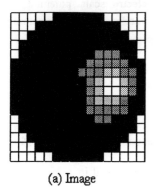

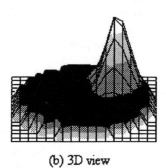

(a) Image   (b) 3D view

Fig. 9   Images produced from an ART algorithm

5. Conclusions

This chapter has presented a general overview of existing inductive EMT systems, concentrating in particular on three examples and has included a description of some of the reconstruction algorithms currently used. The important features of these types of system with respect to other electrical tomographic techniques are:

i.   Non-contacting.
ii.   Provides information on the distribution of conductive and/or magnetic material.
iii.   Ability to operate at high excitation frequencies (i.e. MHz) to provide fast image capture rates.
iv.   Separate excitation and detection coil assemblies which provide flexibility in the design of the sensor array.

At present, these systems are all laboratory based and were developed primarily for feasibility purposes. Consequently, this form of tomography is at a very early stage of development. The initial results from these systems however are promising and it is expected that more practical prototype systems will emerge shortly.

Notation

A	vector magnetic potential	j	$(-1)^{\frac{1}{2}}$
B	magnetic flux density	q	charge density
D	electrical displacement	(r,ϕ)	detector position in circular
E	electric field strength		coordinates
H	magnetic field strength	R	radius of the target object
J	current density	ε	electrical permittivity

μ magnetic permeability of object Φ electric scalar potential
         material $\underline{\nabla}\cdot$ vector divergence operator
σ electrical conductivity of object $\underline{\nabla}\times$ vector curl operator
         material
ω angular frequency

References

[1]   D. C Barber and B. H. Brown: Applied Potential Tomography. J. Phys. E.,
       Sci. Instrum. **17**, pp. 723-733, (1984).

[2]   A. D. Seager, D. C. Barber and B. H. Brown: Electrical impedance imaging.
       IEE Proc. A, pp. 201-210, (1987).

[3]   S. M. Huang, C. G. Xie, R. Thorn, D. Snowden and M. S. Beck: Design of
       sensor electronics for electrical capacitance tomography.   IEE Proc. G, **139**,
       pp. 83-88, (1992).

[4]   C. G. Xie, S. M. Huang, B. S. Hoyle, R. Thorn, C. Lenn, D. Snowden and M.
       S. Beck: Electrical capacitance tomography for flow imaging: system model
       for development of image reconstruction algorithms & design of primary
       sensors. IEE Proc. G, **139**, pp. 89-98 (1992).

[5]   J. M Scaife, R. C. Tozer and I. L. Freeston: Conductivity and permittivity
       images from an induced current electrical impedance tomography system. IEE
       Proc. A., **141**, pp. 356-362, (1994).

[6]   B. Horner and F. Mesch: An induction flowmeter insensitive to asymmetric
       flow profiles. European Concerted Action on Process Tomography conference,
       ISBN 0 9523165 2 8, Bergen, April (1995).

[7]   Y. Tomita and S. Honda: Estimation of velocity profile by magnetic
       flowmeter with rotating field. SICE conference, Kumamoto Japan, pp. 1301 -
       1304, (1992).

[8]   J. H. Moran and K. S. Kunz: Basic theory of induction well logging and
       application to the study of two coil sondes. Geophysics, **XXVII**, pp.829-58,
       (1962).

[9]   M. D. Harpen: Eddy current distribution in cylindrical samples: effects on
       equivalent sample impedance. Phys. Med. Biol., **34**, pp. 1229-38, (1989).

[10]   R. A. Albrechtsen, Z. Z. Yu and A. J. Peyton: Towards an analytical
       approach for determining the sensitivity limits and sensitivity maps of mutual
       inductance tomography. European Concerted Action on Process Tomography
       conference, Bergen, Norway, ISBN 0 9523165 2 8, pp. 288-99, (1995).

[11]   S. Al-Zeibak, N. H. Saunders: A feasibility study of *In Vivo* electromagnetic
       imaging. Phys. Med. Biol., **38**, pp. 151-60, (1993).

[12]   Z. Z. Yu, A. J. Peyton, W. F. Conway, L. A. Xu and M. S. Beck: Imaging
       system based on electromagnetic tomography (EMT). Electronics Letters,
       29(7), pp. 625-26, (1993).

Part II

Reconstruction

Chapter 9

Tomographic Reconstruction

David M. Scott
Du Pont Central Research and Development
E. I. du Pont de Nemours and Co. (Inc.)
Experimental Station, E357
Wilmington, Delaware 19880-0357 USA

1. Definitions

The first section of this book has examined various modalities by which one can probe the interior of a process vessel or pipeline. As discussed in Chapter 2, the interaction of the probe with an industrial process causes a measurable response that depends upon the physical state and distribution of material in the vessel. If the contents, physical state, and distribution are known, then the probe response may be predicted on the basis of well-known physical principles. For example, given a particular spatial distribution of material within a pipeline, one can easily calculate the projection image that would be obtained by radiography. Such a calculation, which is based on a known (or assumed) distribution of material in the pipe, is called a "forward problem" calculation. The task of tomography is to solve the "inverse problem" by determining the material distribution that would give the observed probe responses. In the present example, the task would be analogous to discerning the three-dimensional distribution of material in the pipe by looking at radiographs taken at several different positions around the pipe. Typically, process tomography determines the distribution of material within distinct cross-sectional planes, and a cross-sectional image used to represent the distribution of material. The process of solving the inverse problem to obtain a cross-sectional image is known as "reconstruction". The relationship between the forward problem and the inverse problem (i.e., reconstruction) is more closely examined in the next chapter.

Just as there are many modalities available for probing a process, so there are many reconstruction techniques. Although particular combinations of sensing modality and reconstruction method may be optimal for a given process application, in fact many sensing techniques can be used in conjunction with more than one of the reconstruction approaches discussed below. The premise unifying all tomographic techniques is that the N-dimensional cross sectional image can be reconstructed from several (N-1) dimensional views ("projections") [1].

The concept of a projection is most easily explained in the context of a first-generation x-ray scanner, which scans a collimated x-ray beam along the transverse direction x'. In order to generate a 2-D cross sectional image, a 1-D projection $P_\varphi(x')$ is measured at each orientation angle φ for the object, which has a spatially dependent (2-D) linear attenuation coefficient $\mu(x,y)$ in the measurement plane:

$$P_\varphi(x') = \int \mu(x',y')dy'$$

(1)

Note that the projection has a reduced dimensionality. Here the primed coordinates x' and y' are rotated with respect to the body-fixed coordinates x and y via an orthogonal transformation:

$$\begin{bmatrix} x' \\ y' \end{bmatrix} = \begin{bmatrix} \cos\varphi & -\sin\varphi \\ \sin\varphi & \cos\varphi \end{bmatrix} \cdot \begin{bmatrix} x \\ y \end{bmatrix}$$

(2)

In x-ray tomography these projections are measured at each point (x') from the natural logarithm of the ratio of the incident radiation intensity to the radiation intensity transmitted through the object. This operation linearizes the transmission data and makes it correspond to the projection given in equation (1). Other probing methods may require a different treatment of the projection data.

One way to reconstruct an image of the original object is to "back-project" (replicate) each projection along the direction of y' and to sum all back-projections together. This process is illustrated in Fig. 1, which shows the impulse response of the back-projection reconstruction. Each one of the projections of a point object is a delta function, which is non-zero only at a single point. The back-projection of a point is a line, and the summation over many angles φ is shown in Fig. 1a. Since these projections are 1-D objects, back-projection can be considered as a "smearing" of the projections into a second dimension. The final reconstructed image of the point object is shown in Fig. 1b. This image defines the "point spread function" of the reconstruction.

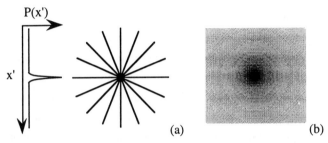

(a)   (b)

Fig. 1 (a) Back-projections of a point are lines (b) Reconstructed image of a point

It is evident from Fig. 1b that images tend to be blurred in this method of reconstruction. Due to the linearity of the imaging process, the reconstructed image of a more complicated object will simply be the superposition of a large number of such blurred points. Although the point spread function for back-projected images is known [2] to have a relatively long-range $1/r$ dependence (where r is the distance from the point), a convolution (filtering) operation performed on the projections before reconstruction improves the image clarity [3]. This approach is the basis of the canonical "filtered back-projection" reconstruction.

Many process tomography methods (most notably the electrical methods) require modifications to the reconstruction procedure just outlined. Electrode arrays that circle pipes generate curved electric fields, so the current paths or capacitive volumes that define the integration paths corresponding to (1) are curved. Thus the back-projections themselves must be curved to match the original electric fields. A more difficult problem is connected with the interaction between the contents of the sensing volume and the electrical field itself. The electrical field is influenced by the composition and distribution of material through which it passes, so the correct placement of the back-projections becomes difficult. This "soft-field" effect may be quite large in some applications, requiring the use of more sophisticated reconstruction algorithms.

2. Approaches to reconstruction

Given the variety of probing techniques, it is to be expected that there are also a wide variety of techniques used for reconstructing cross-sectional images from the projection data. It should be noted that there are several ways to organize these techniques. One review [4] of reconstruction methods used in process tomography classified the major techniques into diffraction, transmission, and electrical categories. The next chapter of this book will present a different classification based on the mathematical representation used to describe the interactions (scalar, vectorial, tensorial), and many other schemes are possible. In order to provide a context for the reconstruction techniques described in the subsequent chapters, we will for the moment consider an overview of the various techniques based on their general approach to the inverse problem. Most tomography reconstruction techniques can be categorized as Direct, Iterative, Model-based, Analog, or Heuristic.

2.1 Direct methods

The direct methods are based on the pioneering work of Radon [1]. These reconstruction methods include the filtered back-projection method outlined above and the central slice method [5] used extensively in computed tomography. Transform methods [6] might also be considered in this category. This type of approach assumes that a full set of projection data is available, and the inverse problem is solved analytically using either a continuous or a discrete implementation. If the projection set is incomplete or noisy, the final image will be distorted by artifacts of the reconstruction process [7,8]. A systematic study of such artifacts was recently undertaken by Müller, who showed [9] that multiple truncated projections (those not "wide enough" to span the width of the object) could be combined to give an error-free reconstruction. This synthetic aperture approach is clearly applicable to the x-ray tomography of large industrial vessels.

In one form or another, backprojection (as described above) is one of the most common reconstruction algorithms. It is widely used in x-ray tomography, and it forms the basis of analog reconstruction techniques as discussed below. Backprojection is also used in applied potential tomography [10] and in capacitance tomography [11].

Historically, tomography has been used to reconstruct single cross sections (two-dimensional images) of an object from 1-D projections. Likewise, many process tomography applications provide images in a single plane (or in a small number of fixed planes). However, direct algorithms [12-14] have been developed over the past 15 years to reconstruct three dimensional volume images from radiographic 2-D projections. The application of these techniques to process tomography has not been fully explored.

2.2 *Iterative methods*

As the name implies, iterative reconstruction techniques solve the inversion problem by comparing the projections of an assumed solution to the projections actually measured, adjusting the assumed solution for a better fit, and repeating the process until the solution converges. A finite element method is generally employed in such calculations. These methods include the optimization approach [15], variations on the Algebraic Reconstruction Technique (ART) [16], and the approach described in Chapter 14.

For example, an iterative technique often employed in Electrical Impedance Tomography (EIT) applications is the Newton-Raphson method [17]. As in any iterative technique, there is an error (the "objective function") to be minimized. In this case the objective function $\Phi(\rho)$ is defined to be

$$\Phi(\rho) = (1/2)(\mathbf{f}(\rho) - \mathbf{V}_0)^T(\mathbf{f}(\rho) - \mathbf{V}_0) \qquad (3)$$

where $\mathbf{V}_0$ is the measured voltage and $\mathbf{f}(\rho)$ represents the estimated voltages based on a resistivity distribution ρ. In order to minimize $\Phi(\rho)$, its first derivative is expanded in a

Taylor series about a point ρ^k and set equal to zero, keeping only the linear terms. Solving for the change in ρ^k, one obtains the the update equation [18]:

$$\Delta\rho^k = \left[\mathbf{f}'(\rho^k)^T \; \mathbf{f}'(\rho^k)\right]^{-1}\left[\mathbf{f}'(\rho^k)\right]^T\!\left[\mathbf{f}(\rho^k) - \mathbf{V}_0\right] \qquad (4)$$

After the resistivity distribution is updated according to (4), the process is repeated until the convergence criterion is met. This algorithm is often used for non-linear problems.

2.3 Model-based methods

Model-based methods assume a specific physical model of the process to be imaged. From the physical model, which includes parameters that describe the spatial distribution of material, one can calculate the interaction of the sensor (x-ray, electrical current, etc.) with the contents of the process. The image can be reconstructed by first using an optimization routine to find the parameters that give the best agreement between the calculated and measured projections [15]. Once the parameter values have been established, the tomographic image can be reconstructed from the model. The optimization component of this approach requires a number of iterations, so these methods may be seen as a sub-set of the iterative methods. This approach to the reconstruction problem is more fully described in Chapter 11.

A model-based reconstruction can be used effectively even when the projection data is noisy or incomplete, because the model allows the substitution of observed (or assumed) information for some of the projection data. Of course, this technique can be applied only if there is sufficient *a priori* knowledge about the system; therefore the approach may work well only for certain applications. Model-based reconstruction methods clearly hold much promise and their use was recently endorsed by participants in a workshop on reconstruction techniques for process tomography [19].

2.4 Analog methods

This approach uses the same theoretical concepts as the direct method, but the implementation is radically different from conventional tomography. In the previous methods, it has been tacitly assumed that the reconstruction process was a set of calculations being carried out on a digital computer (which might be a transputer array). Analog methods, in contrast, use either analog computers or opto-electronic circuits to reconstruct the image. In virtually every case, the reconstruction is actually based on simple back-projection or filtered back-projection. The advantage of using analog methods is that they tend to be faster and less expensive to implement, but the image quality is generally inferior to that of conventional tomography.

One of the earliest analog tomography methods [20] produced an unfiltered back-projection image by placing film in the plane of the x-ray fan beam. As the object and film were rotated synchronously, a tomographic image was produced on the film. Another approach [21] used x-ray film to detect the projection data, and a subsequent back-projection step was needed for the reconstruction. Incoherent optical processors based on optical transfer function synthesis have demonstrate the ability to reconstruct cross-sectional images directly from projection data stored on x-ray film [22]. Other optical devices reconstruct the images directly from projection data provided by x-ray image intensifiers [23]. Optical techniques have also been used to filter the projection data in order to improve the reconstructed images [24]. These optical approaches may be used with the optical tomography techniques discussed in Chapter 7, but in general the use of optical reconstruction does not require the use of optical tomography to provide the projection data.

Tomographic images can also be reconstructed with analog electronic circuits. The author has demonstrated [25, 26] an analog system that reconstructs images directly on the face of a storage oscilloscope. The system implements a filtered backprojection reconstruction by using analog multipliers to rotate the oscilloscope's backprojection synchronously with the rotating projection. The reconstruction appears in real time, regardless of the size of the projection data set. This approach has been shown to be mathematically equivalent to the canonical back-projection algorithm [26]. The quality of the images is adequate for many applications, but it could be improved by filtering the projection data. It has been demonstrated that a tapped analog delay line can filter projection data before reconstruction [27], so a filtered back-projection system can also be implemented entirely with analog electronics. The combination of speed and economy in this approach is particularly relevant in the the context of process tomography.

2.5 *Heuristic methods*

The recent resurgence of interest in neural networks has impacted many fields including process tomography. Neural networks are useful because they offer a heuristic method of relating input signals to output signals for complex systems that cannot be modelled. These networks are essentially based on neural structures found in simple organisms, and they may be either hard-wired or virtual (existing as a program in a computer). Many of the concepts can be traced to the work on perceptrons [28] and to previous research on self-organizing systems [29].

A typical neural network is built from interconnected layers composed of single processing elements ("neurons"). A neuron has many inputs but only one output, which may be connected to other neurons through weighted connections. Thus, the output of a given neuron is based on a nonlinear transformation of the weighted sum of its inputs. The output values of the neurons in the final ("output") layer of the network depend on the pattern of values presented at the input layer. To train the neural network, a series of input patterns are presented, and the output is compared to the "correct" response for that particular input. The weights interconnecting the neurons are changed according to a "learning rule"; the network adapts to its environment by modifying the weights according to this learning rule [30]. The "knowledge" contained in the network is stored in the values of the weights interconnecting the neurons. Therefore, the knowledge is transferrable from one net to another simply by copying the values of the weights.

The application of neural networks to image reconstruction in process tomography is discussed in Chapter 13. A slightly different approach is based on the concept that useful information about a process (such as void fraction or multi-phase flow velocities) may be obtained directly from the projection data without a full reconstruction of the cross-sectional image. This alternative approach has the benefit of faster sampling rates and higher throughput. In addition, the hardware needed to extract pertinent information may be less complex than that needed to reconstruct images. A neural network of this type has been used to identify flow regimes in sand flow [31].

3.   Conclusions

It can be seen from the foregoing that the reconstruction of cross-sectional images may be accomplished in a variety of ways. The best choice depends on the particular process to be imaged and, as pointed out in Chapter 2, the process equipment itself.

The preceding discussion has assumed that the purpose of process tomography is to generate cross sectional images. Strictly speaking, that purpose is the definition of tomography. It should nonetheless be acknowledged that the interest in process tomography comes from a desire to better understand a given chemical process, and that understanding does not necessarily require images. For instance, the use of correlation techniques to obtain flow fields is properly regarded as process tomography, but the flow at any point could be fed into the process controller without generating an image of the flow field. Thus, the utility of these techniques does not necessarily depend on the reconstructed image.

A final point needs to be raised concerning the reconstruction of these images. It is generally assumed that the projection data is free from errors, but in fact the projection data will be noisy, and there may be missing data (due to malfunctioning detectors or truncated projections). Given the reality of imperfect projection data, it is necessary to consider the effect of noise on the reconstructed image within the context of how much error in the image can be tolerated. In the case of transaxial computed tomography, an analysis [32] of the quantum statistics of the radiation source has been used to predict the ultimate performance that can be achieved, and methods have been developed to determine the effects of partial information loss [33]. Chapter 12 of this volume addresses the noise issue within the specific context of process tomography.

References

[1]   J. Radon, Berichte Verh. Sachsische Akad. Wiss., Leipzig, Math. Phys. Kl. **69**:262-7 (1917).

[2]   A. Rosenfeld and A. C. Kak, Digital Picture Processing, 2nd edition (Academic Press, New York, 1982), vol. 1, p. 375.

[3]   H. H. Barrett and W. Swindell, Proc. IEEE **65** 89-107 (1977).

[4]   C. G. Xie, in Proceedings of ECAPT '93, ed. M. S. Beck et al. (UMIST, Manchester, 1994), pp 115-9.

[5]   A. C. Kak and M. Slaney, Principles of Computerized Tomographic Imaging (IEEE Press, New York, 1987).

[6]   R. M. Lewitt, Proc. IEEE **71**:390-408 (1983).

[7]   A. Macovski, Proc. IEEE **71**:373-8 (1983).

[8]   M. Soumekh, IEEE Trans. Acoustics Speech and Signal Processing **ASSP-34**: 952-62 (1986).

[9]   M. Müller, Ph.D. thesis, University of Delaware, 1993.

[10]   D. C. Barber, B. H. Brown, and I. L. Freeston, Elec. Lett. **19**:933-5 (1983).

[11]   G. E. Fasching and N. S. Smith, Rev. Sci. Instrum. **62**:2243-2251 (1991).

[12]   M. Y. Chiu, H. H. Barrett, and R. G. Simpson, J. Opt. Soc. Am. **70**:755-62 (1980).

[13]   L. A. Feldkamp, L. C. Davis, and J. W. Kress, J. Opt. Soc. Am. A **1**:612-9 (1984).

[14]   P. Rizo, P. Grangeat, P. Sire, P. Lemasson, and P. Melennec, J. Opt. Soc. Am. A **8**:1639-48 (1991).

[15]   Ø. Isaksen and J. E. Nordtvedt, Meas. Sci. Technol. **4**:1464-75 (1993).

[16] A. Rosenfeld and A. C. Kak (1982), *op. cit.*, pp. 415-427.

[17] T. J. Yorkey, J. G. Webster, and W. J. Tompkins, Proc. Annu. Int. Conf. IEEE Engineering in Medicine and Biology Society **8**:339-42 (1986).

[18] P. Hua and E. J. Woo, in Electrical Impedance Tomography, ed. J. G. Webster (Adam Hilger, Bristol, 1990), p. 124.

[19] D. M. Scott, in Proceedings of ECAPT '93, ed. M. S. Beck et al. (UMIST, Manchester, 1994), pp 41-4.

[20] W. Watson, U. S. Pat. 2,196,618 (1940); see also A. Lindegaard-Andersen and G. Thuesen, J. Phys. E **11**:805-11 (1978).

[21] G. Frank, U. S. Pat. 2,281,931 (1942).

[22] J. E. Greivenkamp, W. Swindell, A, F. Gmitro, and H. H. Barrett, Applied Optics **20**: 264-73 (1981).

[23] R. J. Gelik, Optica Acta **11**:1367-76 (1979).

[24] H. H. Barrett and W. Swindell, Proc. IEEE **65**:89-107 (1977).

[25] D. M. Scott, in Proceedings of ECAPT '93, ed. M. S. Beck et al. (UMIST, Manchester, 1994), pp 124-7.

[26] D. M. Scott and M. Müller, "Low-Cost Instrument for Real-Time X-Ray Tomography", submitted to Meas. Sci. Technol. (1995).

[27] A. M. Garvie and G. C. Sorell, Rev. Sci. Instrum. **61**:138-45 (1990).

[28] M. Minsky and S. Papert, Perceptrons (MIT Press, Cambridge MA, 1969).

[29] A useful introduction to neural nets is D. E. Rumelhart and J. L. McClelland, Parallel Distributed Processing (MIT Press, Cambridge MA, 1986), vol. 1.

[30]   D. O. Hebb, The Organization of Behavior (Wiley, New York, 1949).

[31]   A. R. Bidin, R. G. Green, M. E. Shackleton, and R. W. Taylor, Part. Part Syst. Charact. **10**: 234-238 (1993).

[32]   H. H. Barrett, T. Bowen, S. K. Gordon, and R. S. Hershel, Computers in Biology and Medicine, **6**:307-23 (1976).

[33]   M. Müller, in Proceedings of ECAPT '94, ed. M. S. Beck et al. (UMIST, Manchester, 1994), pp 234-43.

Chapter 10

Sensing Principles and Reconstruction

F. Mesch
Institut für Meß- und Regelungstechnik
Universität (T.H.) Karlsruhe
Postfach 69 80, D - 76128 Karlsruhe, Germany

. Introduction

The aim of a tomographic system is to have a "look" inside a measurement volume without using probes, i.e. in a non-invasive manner; any sensors may be placed only outside the boundaries of the measurement volume. The signal carrier between the measurand inside and the sensors outside the measurement volume can be constituted by a wide variety of physical quantities; some of them are discussed in the first part of this book. Within the measurement volume, the spatially distributed measurand interacts with the signal carrier such that its amplitude, phase, frequency, propagation time or propagation direction is altered. The signals obtained from the sensors are related to the measurand by complex multidimensional integrals, which is called the *forward problem*. The *inverse problem,* namely determining the measurand from the signals, is called *reconstruction.* Both, the forward and consequently the inverse problem, depend on the physical nature of the signal carrier and its interaction with the measurand. It is the aim of this chapter to review various types of interaction and to try a systematic classification. Based on this classification, some general statements on sensor design will be derived.

. Scalar, vector and tensor fields

Spatially distributed measurands can be viewed as *fields.* Generally in physics, fields are classified into scalar, vector and tensor fields, depending on what type of quantity is assigned to any point in space. Accordingly, the first important criterion for classifying the great number of sensing effects is to distinguish between scalar vectorial and tensorial interaction between measurand and signal carrier.

The existing literature on tomography almost exclusively deals with scalar in teraction. Examples of scalar fields are any potentials, temperature fields, or distribu tions of densities, of disperse phases, of chemical compositions and the like. The per tinent mechanisms of interaction with the signal carrier may be subdivided into ab sorption, emission, scattering, diffraction, reflection, variation of electrical imped ances, fluorescence, nuclear resonance - there are certainly some others more.

In contrast to scalar fields, tomography of vector and tensor fields is quite a new topic. Examples of vector fields interesting for process applications are velocity dis tributions of flowing fluids, gradients of space-dependent refractive index, or elec tromagnetic fields. An important example of a tensor field is mechanical stress distri bution. Pertinent sensing effects will be discussed in connection with the application examples in Section 2.2.

2.1 Some theoretical results for vector tomography

Before going into details, some general statements can be made concerning principal limitations in reconstructing vector and tensor fields, depending on the type of interaction. According to Helmholtz's decomposition theorem, any vector field $\vec{f}(\vec{r})$ may be expressed as the sum of an "irrotational component" $\vec{f_1}(\vec{r})$ and a "solenoidal component" $\vec{f_2}(\vec{r})$

$$\vec{f}(\vec{r}) = \vec{f_1}(\vec{r}) + \vec{f_2}(\vec{r}). \quad (1)$$

The irrotational component is defined by curl $\vec{f_1}(\vec{r}) = \vec{0}$ and will thus be called here "curl-free component", the solenoidal component is defined by

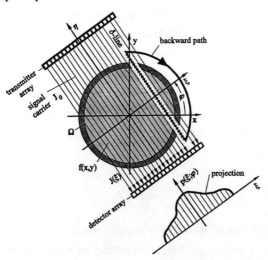

Fig. 1: Parallel projection and contour integration

div $\vec{f_2}(\vec{r}) = 0$ and will be called "source-free component". Consider now a typical parallel projection as discussed in [1, 2] and as shown here in Fig. 1. The interaction between the object $\vec{f}(\vec{r})$ and the signal carrier within the measuring volume Ω is assumed to be described by *line* integrals. The integral along the δ-line in Fig. 1 is now complemented by an integration path backwards outside the measuring volume (or along its boundary), assuming the field there to be zero such that the backward path does not contribute to the integral. In this simple way, a closed *contour* integral is formed, and the integral theorems of Gauss and Stokes and - more generally - the methods of field theory and vector analysis may be applied. Using this theory, it was shown in [3-5] that one must distinguish between two types of interaction:

- longitudinal interaction where only the field component in the direction of wave propagation of the signal carrier is measured
- transverse interaction where only the field component perpendicular to the wave propagation is measured.

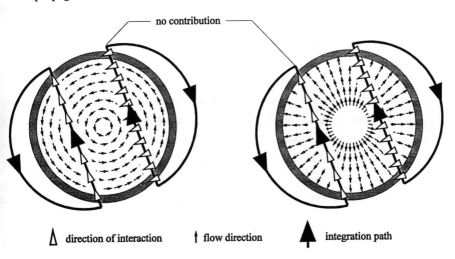

Fig. 2: Vortex field (left) and source field (right) and integration paths with longitudinal and transversal interaction

The longitudinal interaction yields only the source-free component, and the transverse interaction only the curl-free component. This theoretical result may be visualized without formulae by Fig. 2; on the left a pure vortex field, on the right a pure source field is shown, and in each figure one integration path with longitudinal and another one with transversal interaction is indicated. By simple symmetry considerations, one can confirm the above statements. Thus a complete reconstruction of a general vector field is possible only if both interactions are available. In practice, however, ofter only one type of interaction is physically possible, as will be shown in the next sec-tion. Then one must rely on the a-priori knowledge that only one field componen* exists.

Difficulties further arise in the case of non-vanishing boundary conditions. This can be made clear also from Fig. 1. There it had been assumed that the backward path does not contribute to the integral; in other words, the field must vanish at is bounda-ries, as is usually the case for boundaries at infinity. With boundaries constituted by the walls of a pipe, however, one has to be careful; a flow field, for example, will be zero at the wall, but a temperature field will not. In the latter case, reconstruction is directly possible by ART, but more involved when using Fourier transform [5].

For tensor fields, the theory is considerably more complex; the basic results are analogous to those given for vector tomography [6].

2.2 *Examples of vector tomography*

Fig. 3 schematically shows the velocity field of a flowing fluid, together with a system for measuring travelling times between ultrasonic transducer arrays. Consider two single transducers A and B; first A is used as a transmitter and B as a receiver, and the time-of-flight τ_{AB} from A to B is measured, and then with B transmitting and A receiving, τ_{BA} in the opposite direction is measured. Since the resulting propagation velocity of sound in a moving medium is the superposition of the sound velocity in a static medium and the local flow velocity, the sound speed c may be obtained from the sum

$$\tau_{AB} + \tau_{BA} = 2\int_A^B \frac{1}{c(\vec{r})}\,d\,r \qquad (2)$$

and the local flow velocity $\vec{v}$ from the difference

$$\tau_{AB} - \tau_{BA} = 2\int_A^B \frac{\vec{v}(\vec{r})\cdot\vec{i}}{c^2(\vec{r})}\,d\,r, \qquad (3)$$

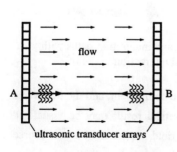

Fig. 3: Ultrasonic time-of-flight measurement

where $v \ll c$ and small local variations of c have been assumed, where $\int...d r$ are line integrals etween A and B, and where $\vec{t}$ is a unit vector in the direction of sound wave propagation. Eq. (2) represents a scalar interaction, and since c depends on temperature, it may be used to determine the temperature distribution in flames [7]. Eq. (3) represents a longitudinal vectorial interaction; in [4] it has been used to measure flow velocity fields of water in an arrangement similar to Fig. 3, and in [7] it was used to measure flow velocity fields in a furnace.

It is physically obvious that the system of Fig. 3 would completely fail with the source field of Fig. 2 right (which one could imagine to be the flow in a basin produced by a fountain in its centre). So source fields require a sensor system with transversal interaction. A conceivable solution is indicated in Fig. 4; there, the ultrasonic beam generated by transmitter A is assumed to be deflected by the transverse flow. However, this solution has (to the author's knowledge) not yet been verified experimentally. It should be noted that even in the absence of literal sources of mass flow, a compressible flow is not "source-free" in the sense of vector analysis. So when applying time-of-flight measurements to gas flows where density variations might occur, care should be taken.

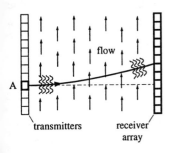

Fig. 4: Deflection of ultrasonic rays

In another example just these density variations are measured. Fig. 5 shows a classical optical Schlieren system. A first lens generates a parallel beam of (incoherent) light, where the phase object with space-dependent refractive index n is placed. In the Fourier plane of the second lens a knife-edged stop is so adjusted that - without object - only half of the light beam can pass via a field lens to a CCD-camera. Variations of n cause deflections of the light beam resulting in intensity variations of the detected light. It may be shown [8, 9] that the resulting normalized intensity variation is

$$\frac{\Delta I}{I} = K \int (\vec{t} \times \vec{b}) \cdot \mathrm{grad}\,(\ln n)\, \mathrm{d}\,r \quad (4)$$

where the unit vectors $\vec{t}$ and $\vec{b}$ are

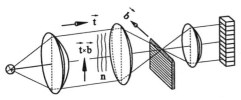

Fig. 5: Schlieren system for measuring
refractive index

defined in Fig. 5 and where $\int ...d\vec{r}$ is a line integral in direction of $\vec{t}$. The vector product $\vec{t} \times \vec{b}$ is a unit vector normal to $\vec{t}$ and $\vec{b}$, i.e. in vertical direction in Fig. 5. Therefore only the gradient component in this direction is measured, which means a transverse vectorial interaction. It is interesting to note that also none of the other well-known optical methods for flow visualization shows a longitudinal vectorial interaction; shadowing, Moiré and shearographic methods have transverse vectorial interaction, whereas interferometric methods have scalar interaction [9]. So with these methods, one must rely on the a-priori information that the fields to be measured are curl-free which is satisfied for the case of refractive index gradients. In [8, 9], the Schlieren system of Fig. 5 has been rotated relative to a flame, and by tomographic methods, the refractive index field was reconstructed from which temperature distributions have been computed.

3. Signal carrier and types of integrals

The next important criterion for classifying sensing effects is the type of integrals describing them mathematically. This point of view, of course, relies on the assumption that the interaction between measurand and signal carrier along its way through the measuring volume can be modelled by integrals, which indeed is mostly the case, apart from inherently discrete effects occurring at singular points in space, as specular reflection of ultrasound from particles [10], or as positron emission.

Computer tomography started from absorption of X-rays in medical applications, which can adequately be described by line integrals along parallel, straight integration paths. The theory based on this model led to the well-known analytical tools for reconstruction, as Radon's inversion formula, backprojection, and Fourier slice theorem [1, 2]. Also the examples discussed in Section 2.2 led to line integrals Eqs. (2) - (4).

Other signal carriers and other interaction mechanisms, however, often require different models; the differences concern especially the geometry of integration domain. Another important complication is called the "soft field effect" which means that the spatial distribution of the exciting signal carrying field is affected by the measurand resulting in a highly nonlinear sensing effect. Although these two issues are partly interrelated, they will be discussed separately in the following sections.

.1 Integration domain

The simplest deviation from the parallel-ray model of Fig. 1 occurs if a point source rather than a line source is used generating a fan beam instead of a parallel beam. For this case still analytical reconstruction formulae exist [2]. A more severe deviation is the bending of rays caused by refraction effects; although the interaction is still described by line integrals, the curvature of the integration path depends on the result of the reconstruction, and no analytical methods exist. The practical approach is an iteration procedure where first a reconstruction is computed neglecting refraction, which is then corrected in subsequent steps.

If the signal carrier is a wave with a wavelength comparable to or even larger than the sizes of the local inhomogeneities of the measurand, the wave is scattered into all directions. For this case, there exists a special analytical model called diffraction tomography [2]. Process applications are discussed in [11].

So far, waves have been considered as signal carrier, propagating from transmitters to detectors. Now quite another type of signal carrier will be considered, namely quasistatic electromagnetic fields. These fill the space between electrodes or poles and therefore lead to volume integrals. Two different types of systems will be considered.

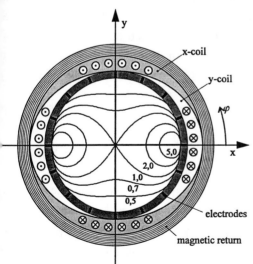

Fig. 6: Inductive flow meter

Fig. 6 shows a novel inductive flowmeter. Consider first the pair of y-coils and the pair of x-electrodes which form a conventional inductive flowmeter. The voltage induced between the electrodes is given by the volume integral

$$u = \iiint_\Omega (\vec{B} \times \vec{W}) \cdot \vec{v} \, d^3x \qquad (5)$$

where $\vec{v}$ is the local flow velocity, $\vec{B}$ the magnetic induction, and $\vec{W}$ a weight function corresponding to

the Green's function describing the configuration of point electrodes; its modulus i[
two dimensions is depicted within the pipe. Assuming $\vec{B}$ and $\vec{W}$ to have n[
components in direction of the pipe axis, the vector product $\vec{B} \times \vec{W}$ has onl[
components in this direction. If the coil is wound in such a way that it produces [
current density (= "ampere turns") proportional to $\sin\varphi$, $\vec{B}$ becomes homogeneou[
Nevertheless such flowmeters suffer from errors if the flow profile is not axiall[
symmetric. Therefore this flowmeter is being extended and developed in tw[
directions. Adding a second pair of x-coils, and feeding both coil pairs with tw[
voltages with a phaseshift of 90°, a two-phase system is formed as known fron[
electric machines, generating a rotating magnetic field. Adding also another pair of y
electrodes, one can show [12] that errors in measuring the mean flow rate are reduce[
considerably. Alternatively, if more electrodes are added and their signals evaluate[
by tomographic methods, a reconstruction of the flow profile is possible [13].

Another type of systems is shown in Fig. 7 representing schematically Electric
Impedance Tomography (EIT) that has gained special importance in process tomography. *Impedance* stands either for resistance, capacitance or mutal inductance. In the
first case, the electrodes are in contact with the flow which is assumed to be a conductive liquid, and by measuring the resistance between all possible pairs of electrodes, one aims at measuring any inhomogeneous spatial distribution of conductivity
σ. In the second case, one measures similarly the capacitances between electrodes to[
determine the distribution of permittivity ε in an insulating fluid. In the third case, the
poles represent magnetic excitation and detection coils, and the mutual inductances
are measured to determine the distribution of permeability μ. The basic physical
relations describing these three cases are, respectively:

$$\vec{J} = \sigma \cdot \vec{E}, \quad \vec{D} = \varepsilon \cdot \vec{E}, \quad \vec{B} = \mu \cdot \vec{H} \quad (6)$$

where $\vec{J}$-current density, $\vec{E}$-electrical field, $\vec{D}$-dielectric polarisation, $\vec{B}$-magnetic induction, $\vec{H}$-magnetic field. Since these equations have identical forms, it suffices to calculate the impedance between two electrodes for the case of capacitances. The energy of an electric field is given by

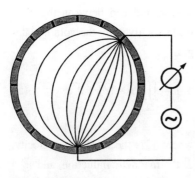

Fig. 7: EIT system

$$W_e = \tfrac{1}{2} \iiint \vec{D}\vec{E}\, d^3x = \tfrac{1}{2} \iiint \varepsilon \left|\vec{E}\right|^2 d^3x. \tag{7}$$

Equating with the energy stored in a capacitance C by voltage u

$$W_e = \frac{1}{2}Cu^2 \tag{8}$$

results in [14]:

$$C = \frac{1}{u^2} \iiint \varepsilon \cdot |\vec{E}|^2 \, d^3x \tag{9}$$

which again is a volume integral. It is quite obvious that this fact has a profound effect on the spatial resolution. Wheras in Fig. 1 each pair of elements of the transmitter/detector arrays generates a signal depending only on the line integral along a thin ray, in Figs. 6 and 7 the whole volume between two electrodes contributes to the signal, which severely limits the possible resolution. A further snag is the inhomogeneous sensitivity. The weight function in Fig. 6 has maxima at the electrode locations, which means the sensitivity is high near the pipe wall and small in the centre. The same is true in Fig. 7 where field lines have been sketched; the sensitivity function is quite similar fo that of Fig. 6 (see e.g. [14]).

3.2   The soft field effect

Although both systems of Figs. 6 and 7 are described by electromagnetic fields, there are some principal differences. The *electromagnetic induction system* of Fig. 6 generates a voltage and might therefore be called *active*. The voltage is a perfect linear function Eq. (5) of the measurand $\vec{v}$, and the measurand does not retroact on the field B. Due to this fact, the number of independent measurements available for tomographic reconstruction equals simply the number of electrodes, if the magnetic field is assumed homogeneous. The number of independent measurements can thus be further increased only with inhomogeneous fields. What types of inhomogeneity were preferable, is not yet clear [13].

The *impedance system* of Fig. 7 must be excited by voltages or currents and might therefore be called passive. The main difference now is that the field generated by these voltages or currents also depends on the distribution of σ, ε or μ, if th' distribution is not uniform. Since the aim of EIT is to image just this distribution, it i always non-uniform. Mathematically therefore, in Eq. (9) one must write $\vec{E} = \vec{E}(\varepsilon$. and a highly non-linear relation results. The impact on reconstruction is that - at lea: in principle - one must use iterative procedures, as already indicated in Sec. 3.1 for th case of bent rays. Another impact is on the question how many independen measurements are possible. Since N electrodes can be combined into

$$n = N(N-1)/2 \tag{10}$$

different pairs, in the pertinent literature it is tacitly assumed that this is also the num ber of independent measurements. Though there are discrepancies. In Electrica Capacitance Tomography (ECT), one usually measures the capacity between two electrodes at one time, as indicated in Fig. 7. In Electrical Resistance Tomography (ERT) however, usually a current is injected in two electrodes and resulting voltage: are measured between pairs of other electrodes, so the electrodes can be combined to

$$n = 6 \binom{N}{4} \tag{11}$$

quadruples of electrodes. In Electro-Magnetic inductance Tomography (EMT) like- wise two coils are excited and another pair of coils are used as search coils. No expla- nation could be found in the literature why the measurement strategies differ between ECT and ERT/EMT.

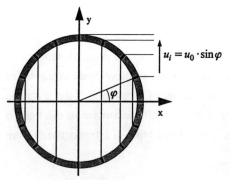

Fig. 8: ECT system with uniform excitation field

Recently, two different approaches for combining and exciting electrodes have been proposed. In [15], instead of pairing single electrodes, various num- bers of electrodes are connected in parallel to form a single electrode, result- ing in an increased number of combina- tions. In [16] and [17], all electrodes are fed simultaneously by voltages being proportional to their geometrical dis- tance, as shown in Fig. 8 for ECT, which results in an approximately homogeneous field. The argument is that the sensitivity in the centre of the pipe is increased, and the over-emphasis in the vicinity of the walls is avoided. In addition, this homogeneous field can easily be rotated by assigning the angle $\varphi = 0$ to other electrodes, analogous to the rotating magnetic field of Fig. 6. It seems to be not yet clear, however, if also the spatial resolution is increased in this way. Also the impact on reconstruction was not yet discussed in the literature. The parallel field lines of Fig. 8 are geometrically similar to Fig. 1, which might induce to use line integrals. This is, however, certainly not possible, because only the exciting field (for $\varepsilon = $ const) is uniform. The real object field, however, is quite different, as sketched in Fig. 9; obviously an object with different ε affects the capacity between several pairs of electrodes, and not only between one pair which would correspond to the line integrals of Fig. 1.

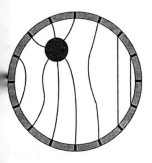

Fig. 9: Real object field

In EIT, for reconstruction one usually neglects the soft field effect. However, to answer the question which combination of electrodes and what measurement strategy is optimal, the nonlinear problem should be solved. Perhaps theoretical methods and approximations such as reviewed in [18] could show the way for an approach. In conclusion, the theory of EIT seems to need further development to give a deeper understandig and to improve sensitivity, accuracy and resolution. In contrast, the theory of electromagnetic induction is much simpler as the phenomenon is linear, and is therefore better developed. A better theory, of course, has also a direct impact on reconstruction. So in [13] specially tailored series expansions of the measurand are proposed. Better theoretical models further allow to include a-priori information in reconstruction, which to a certain extent can compensate for the small number of measurements available [19].

4. Acknowledgement

Fig. 1 (partially) and Fig. 5 have been reproduced from [20] with kind permission by IMEKO.

5. References

[1] D.M. Scott, in this volume.

[2] A.C. Kak, M. Slaney, Principles of Computerized Tomographic Imaging (IEEE Press, New York, 1988).

[3] H. Braun, A. Hauck, IEEE Trans. Signal Proc. 39(1991), pp. 464-471.

[4] A. Hauck, Tomographie von Vektorfeldern, (Fortschritt-Berichte Reihe 8 Nr. 220, VDI-Verlag, Düsseldorf 1990).

[5] A. Trächtler, Tomographie von Vektorfeldern, Teil III (Report 6/1993, Institut für Meß- und Regelungstechnik, Karlsruhe).

[6] A. Trächtler, in Proc. of XIII IMEKO World Congress, Torino 1994, pp. 1893-1898.

[7] A. Schwarz, in Proc. of ECAPT '92, ed. M.S. Beck et al. (Computational Mechanics Publ., Southampton, 1993), pp. 381-389.

[8] A. Schwarz, in Proc. of ECAPT '93, ed. M.S. Beck et al. (UMIST, Manchester, 1994), pp. 293-295.

[9] A. Schwarz, Multitomographische Temperaturmessung in Flammen mit einem Schlierenmeßaufbau (Fortschritt-Berichte Reihe 8 Nr. 444, VDI-Verlag, Düsseldorf 1995).

[10] M.A. Seiraffi, Ultraschall-Computer-Tomographie zur Messung von Zweiphasenströmungen. (Fortschritt-Berichte Reihe 8 Nr. 327, VDI-Verlag, Düsseldorf, 1993).

[11] T.C. Wedberg, J.J. Stamnes, in Proc. of ECAPT '95, ed. M.S. Beck et al. (UMIST, Manchester, 1995), pp. 118-126.

[12] B. Horner, F. Mesch, in Proc. of ECAPT '95 (as [11]), pp. 321-330.

[13] A. Trächtler, A. Wernsdörfer, in this volume.

[14] Q. Chen, B.S. Hoyle, H.J. Strangeways, in Proc. of ECAPT '92 (as [7]), pp. 205-212.

[15] N. Reinecke, D. Mewes, in Proc. of ECAPT '94, ed. M.S. Beck et al. (UMIST, Manchester, 1994), pp. 50-59.

[16] W.Q.Yang et al., in Proc. of ECAPT '95 (as [11]), pp. 266-275.

[17] Z.Z. Yu et al., in Proc. of ECAPT '95 (as [11]), pp. 311-320.

[18] M. Füg, Korrelative Durchfluß-Messung an Zweiphasen-Strömungen mit optischen und kapazitiven Sensoren, (Fortschritt-Berichte Reihe 8 Nr. 217, VDI-Verlag, Düsseldorf, 1990).

[19] A. Wernsdörfer, Tomographische Rekonstruktion von Vektorfeldern mit reduzierten Meßdatensätzen, (Fortschritt-Berichte Reihe 8 Nr. 454, VDI-Verlag, Düsseldorf, 1995).

[20] F. Mesch, as [6], pp. 817-826.

Chapter 11

Test of a Model-Based Reconstruction Algorithm

Ø. Isaksen
Department of Industrial Instrumentation
Christian Michelsen Research
P.O. Box 3, N-5036 Fantoft, Bergen, Norway

1. Introduction

Compared to medical tomography, process tomography differs in two respects. Firstly, the number of sensors possible to fit around the process to be imaged is often low in process tomography, and hence, the number of measurements is low. The reason for this is that, in contradistinction to medical tomography where the patient often is placed inside the tomograph, an ECT or EIT process tomograph must be connected directly to the process to be imaged. Secondly, the sensor techniques used in medical tomography are often "hard-field" sensors. A "hard-field" sensor system sets up a uniform field for which the sensitivity (*i.e.* the change in the measurable parameter as a consequence of a change in the parameter of interest) is independent of the parameter distribution inside the sensor. Many process tomographs are based on "soft-field" sensors (as discussed in the previous chapter). These sensors generate a non-homogeneous field, and the sensitivity distribution inside the field changes as the parameter distribution changes. Due to this characteristic, the commonly used reconstruction algorithms developed for medical tomography (backprojection, filtered backprojection, ART, etc.) cannot be implemented into a "soft-field" sensor system with the same success as for a "hard-field" sensor system.

In this paper a capacitance tomography system will be used to illustrate the above described problem. Also a possible solution to the problem will be outlined and results both from pipe flow imaging and separator interface imaging will be presented.

2.   A capacitance tomography system

A capacitance based imaging system (see Fig. 1) consists of a number of electrodes mounted around the process of interest. By combination $n(n-1)/2$ independent measurements result, where n is the number of electrodes. The measured capacitance between two electrodes is dependent on the dielectric constant of the medium between the two electrodes. Hence, a capacitance tomography system can be used to visualise the medium distribution inside the sensors as long as the distribution consists of components which differs in the dielectric constant.

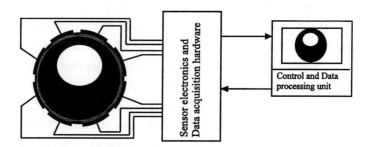

Figure 1. A capacitance tomography system consists of a number of electrodes mounted around the process to be imaged. The data-acquisition unit measures all the capacitances and gives them as input to the reconstruction unit which converts (*i.e.* reconstructs) the measurements to information which describes the distribution inside the pipe.

Capacitance sensors are "soft-field" sensors, and in addition the number of sensors possible to fit around *e.g.* the pipe is low due to the limitation in the sensor electronics. This leads to a challenging reconstruction problem, and is discussed next.

3.   Reconstruction of capacitance data

In this section the performance of the common used Linear Back Projection (LBP) algorithm will be discussed, and an alternative approach named MOdel based Reconstruction (MOR) will be outlined.

3.1.   Linear back projection algorithm

The LBP-algorithm was the first used algorithm to reconstruct capacitance data [1], and still this algorithm is the most commonly used reconstruction technique for capacitance based tomography. Fig. 5c) shows a reconstruction of a stratified distribution based the LBP-algorithm. As can be seen from Fig. 5 the weakness of the LBP-algorithm is that the algorithm smears out sharp transitions in the dielectric constant. This effect is also present when the LBP-algorithm is used together with a "hard-field" sensor (*e.g.* γ-ray) [2], but for a such sensor system it is possible to introduce a correction procedure compensating for this phenomena [2]. It is, however, not possible to realise this correction procedure for a "soft-field" sensor due to the fact that the blurring effect will be dependent on both position inside the cross section and the medium distribution in it self. Therefore, to improve the contrast between the liquid and gas interface some form of thresholding procedure has been applied to the estimated greylevels. Different thresholding procedures have been tested [3,4], non of them being flow regime independent.

In the past few years several attempts have been done to improve the reconstruction [5,6,7,8,9,10,11,12,13]. One of these attempts has been named MOdel based Reconstruction (MOR), and is outlined next.

3.2.   Model based reconstruction

The system model for a capacitance tomography system is based on the Poisson's equation given by:

$$\nabla \cdot \left(\varepsilon(\bar{x})\nabla\Phi\right) = -\rho(\bar{x}), \tag{1}$$

where $\varepsilon(\bar{x})$ is the dielectric constant distribution, Φ is the potential and ρ is the charge distribution. The electric field is given by

$$E = -\nabla\Phi \qquad (2)$$

By applying Gauss law, the induced charge at electrode j when i is the source electrode can be calculated by the following expression:

$$Q_{ij} = \oint_{\Gamma_j} \varepsilon(\vec{x})\vec{E}\cdot\hat{n}dl , \qquad (3)$$

where Γ_j is a closed curve enclosing the detector electrode and $\hat{n}$ is the unit normal vector to Γ_j. Given the charge, Q_{ij}, the capacitance between electrode i and j, C_{ij}, can be calculated by:

$$C_{ij} = \frac{Q_{ij}}{U_{ij}} , \qquad (4)$$

where U_{ij} is the voltage between the source (i) and the detector electrode (j).

Eq. (1) to (4) relates the dielectric constant distribution, $\varepsilon(\vec{x})$, to the measured capacitances, C_{ij}. That is, for a given medium distribution, $\varepsilon(\vec{x})$, and boundary conditions, the capacitances can be calculated by using the equations above.

The inverse problem, which is relevant in reconstructing capacitance data, is to estimate $\varepsilon(\vec{x})$ on the basis of a set of measured capacitances. There exists no explicit expression relating the dielectric constant distribution, $\varepsilon(\vec{x})$, to the measured capacitances. Hence, an implicit solution of the problem must be used.

The number of unknowns to be reconstructed should ideally be less than the number of independent measurements available (28 for an 8-electrode system). One could achieve this by reducing the number of pixels in the LBP-algorithm. However, due to the fact that the number of measurements in a capacitance tomography system is low, the number of pixels must be low, resulting in a poor resolution. In addition the smearing effect in the LBP-algorithm will still be a present phenomena independent of the number of pixels chosen. Keeping in mind that there often will be physical constraints describing situations likely to occur in a process, an alternative approach could be to incorporate *a priori* knowledge of the distribution to be imaged into the reconstruction process. Assume that the process/distribution could be described by n parameters. The MOR-algorithm will then determine the values of those n parameters which given as input to a capacitance simulator, capable of calculating the capacitances as a function of the dielectric distribution inside the sensors, results in minimum discrepancy between measured and simulated capacitances. This could be achieved by using a scheme as illustrated in Fig. 2.

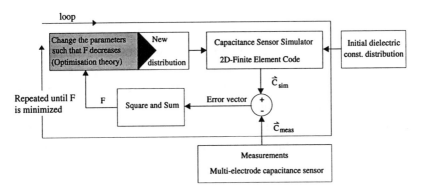

Figure 2. A principal diagram for the MOdel based Reconstruction (MOR) algorithm. This algorithm estimates the dielectric constant distribution which given as input to the sensor simulator result in minimum discrepancy between the measured and simulated capacitance's.

The main parts of the MOR-algorithm are:

- *a parameter representation* of the dielectric constant distribution inside the cross section. The parameterization used to represent the distribution is application dependant. In general it could be stated that the number of parameters describing the distribution must not exceed the number of measurements. For all practical purposes the number of parameters must be kept considerable lower than the number of measurements [14]

- *a capacitance sensor model* capable of calculating the capacitances for a given sensor construction and a parameter representation of the dielectric constant distribution. The capacitance sensor model is based on the Eq. (1) to (4). In this work Eq. (1) has been solved using finite element method.

- *an optimisation routine* minimising the discrepancy between the measured and simulated capacitances. For the reconstructions shown in this paper the Levenberg-Marquardt algorithm has been used [6].

The strength of this approach is that the nature of the capacitance sensors (*e.g.* "soft-field" effects and non-homogenous sensitivity distribution) are fully incorporated into the reconstruction, and that the dielectric constant distribution inside the cross section can be represented by a small number of parameters. This will be illustrated in the nest section.

4.   Test of a model based reconstruction algorithm

The MOR-algorithm has been tested for two different applications; pipe flow imaging [4,6,8,12,13] and oil/water/gas separator imaging [7]. For these two applications it will be possible to obtain parameterization describing the dielectric constant distribution inside the pipe and separator within a reasonable accuracy.

4.1.   Pipe flow imaging

The need for tomographic imaging of multicomponent flow is closely related to problems of measuring flow-velocity, fraction and distribution of individual flow-medium components. Several flow-rate measurement principles are based on the assumption that the flow consists of only one component. Other principles can be applied when several component and/or phases are present, but these principles often require information about the component distribution and how they flow in relation to each other. Such flow regime information can be identified by means of tomographic imaging.

In liquid/gas pipe flow different distribution patterns (*i.e.* flow regimes) can occur, and some of them are shown in Fig. 3. As can be seen it is possible, by approximation, to define a parameterization which represents/describes the different flow regimes reasonably accurate using only a few parameters.

The parameterization shown in Fig. 4a) is based on two parameters, θ and d [12], and can be used to represent stratified, wavy stratified, elongated bubble flow and slug flow regimes (see Fig. 3d)-g)). The parameterization shown in Fig. 4b) is based on three parameters; co-ordinates, (x,y), for the centre of the gas volume and the gas volume radius r [12]. This parameterization can represent slug and annular flow (see Fig. 3b)-c)). Fig. 4c) shows a parameterization based on five parameters, four parameters for describing the ellipse shape and position, and one parameter for describing the amount of gas present in the oil phase [13], ε_{mix} (ε_{mix}, is the dielectric constant for the oil/gas mixture) [15,16]. This parameterization can be used for describing the same type of flow regimes as the parameterization shown in Fig. 4b), but in addition a more flexible gas phase shape and gas bubbles in the oil phase can described by specifying (a,b) and ε_{mix}, respectively.

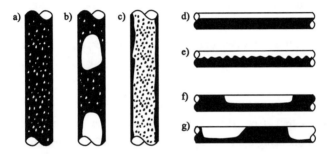

Figure 3. Common flow regimes in a liquid/gas pipe flow. In vertical pipe flow; a) bubble flow, b) slug flow and c) annular flow. In horizontal pipe flow; d) stratified flow, e) stratified wavy flow, f) elongated bubble flow and g) slug flow.

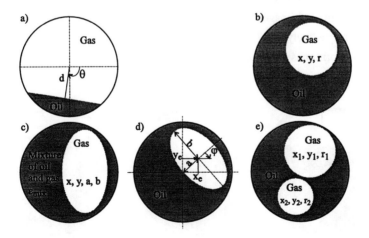

Figure 4. Different parameterization of the flow regimes. a) Stratified distributions, b) Circular gas phase (*e.g.* annular flow), c) Circular or elliptical shaped gas phase surrounded by a mixture of oil and gas, d) Stratified or elliptical/circular flow regimes, and e) Gas bubble flow regime.

Also a parameterization capable of representing both a bubble, slug and stratified distributions is possible to realize, see Fig. 4d). This parameterization is based on five parameters, four parameters for describing the position and form of the ellipse and one angle parameter [6]. Obviously ε_{mix} could be added as the 6th parameter to enable representation of gas in the oil phase.

The flow regime shown in Fig. 3a), *i.e.* small gas bubbles dispersed into the oil phase, must be represented using a number of bubbles or by using the ε_{mix} parameter. As the gas bubbles becomes small and immense in number the bubble parameterization becomes impractical. Two gas bubbles have been the maximum number tested in this work (see Fig. 4e)) [13]. However, a gas fraction measurement, ε_{mix}, will be sufficient for the majority of applications.

Fig. 5 shows a reconstruction based on an 8-electrode capacitance pipe flow tomography system (see Fig. 1). The capacitance measurements have been reconstructed both using the LBP-algorithm and the MOR-algorithm. Air and oil have been used to form the regime for which the oil fraction equals *0.750*. For this case the MOR-algorithm is based on an ellipse parameterization as shown in Fig. 4d). Clearly it can be seen that the MOR-algorithm reconstructs the distribution more accurately than the LBP-algorithm. Due to the smoothing effect in the LBP-image it is difficult to decide where the oil/air interface is located. The calculated oil fraction on the basis of the reconstructed images in Fig. 5 is *0.740* and *0.675* for the MOR- and LBP-algorithm, respectively [8]. This means that the error in the fraction estimate based on the MOR-algorithm is *1.3%*, and *10%* for the LBP-algorithm.

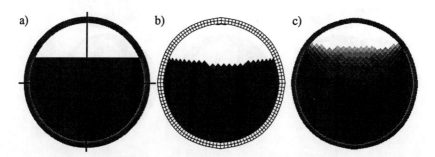

Figure 5. Reconstruction of a stratified distribution with γ = *0.750*. a) The experimental situation. b) Reconstructed by the MOR-algorithm. c) Reconstruction based on the LBP-algorithm.

4.2. Separator imaging

The quality of the product that leaves a water/oil/gas separator is determined by the separator design and control. Current control strategies for separators are extremely simple due to lack of reliable interface level measurement system. At Chr. Michelsen Research (CMR) there has been developed a capacitance based tomography system for interface imaging inside a separator, see Fig. 6 [7]. The tomography system consists of a capacitance sensor system, data acquisition system, and a MOR-algorithm implemented on a personal computer.

This type of application of a capacitance tomography system has strict demands to the accuracy in the reconstruction algorithm. As illustrated in Fig. 5c), the LBP algorithm smears out sharp transitions between areas of different dielectric constants and cannot be used in this case. By using the MOR-algorithm, the interfaces inside an oil/water/gas separator can be imaged. For this case the different interface heights can be used as parameters to be reconstructed. This is an example of the usefulness in incorporation *a priori* information into the reconstruction process. There is no need for *e.g.* having the flexibility in the reconstruction algorithm to image a situation where the oil is beneath the water phase, simply because it will never happen.

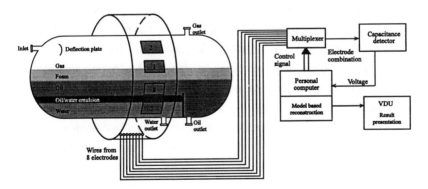

Figure 6. A tomography system for imaging the interface levels inside an oil/water/gas separator. The capacitance sensor consists of 8-electrodes (25 cm long) mounted symmetrically around the separator, and an earthed screen surrounding the electrodes to avoid interference from external fields. The measurements are done sequentially. The PC controls the multiplexer to select a certain electrode pair, and the capacitance detector is used to measure the capacitance. The personal computer reads the measured capacitance into the computer memory, and repeat the process until all measurements are taken. The measurements are then given as input to the reconstruction algorithm which transform the measurements to interface levels.

The measurement system has been installed on a plexiglas separator ($\emptyset = 1\ m$) which was connected to a flow-rig at CMR. The results from the separator tomograph were displayed on a computer screen both by numbers and by an image.

The system can potentially measure the water, oil/water emulsion, oil, and foam heights inside a separator on a process plant. So far, however, the tomograph has been tested for on-line imaging of water, oil, and air interface levels (during water/oil/air tests) and for oil, foam, and air interface imaging (during oil/air tests). The obtained accuracy is within 1.0 cm for all phases. The tomograph also detected the presence of foam.

5.   Conclusions

A model based reconstruction algorithm has been presented. Test results for two different applications (pipe flow and water/oil/gas separator imaging) have been shown. For pipe flow imaging the algorithm has so far been tested for off-line reconstruction of measurements on static flow regimes. The flow regimes have been reconstructed using different parameter representations. The MOR-algorithm has been compared with the commonly used LBP-algorithm, and it is evident that the MOR-algorithm lead to better quality in the reconstruction. The results obtained have been compared with the actual ("true") dielectric constant distribution, and the results prove that the MOR-algorithm represents a step towards quantitative capacitance based tomography. The convergence towards the solution has been tested for different initial distributions [12,13], and it is often observed that the convergence time is dependent on the chosen initial distribution. However, in a real implementation of a tomography system based on the MOR-algorithm the initial distribution will be chosen equal to the previous solution. This strategy was used during the separator tomography work, and represented an efficient approach for choosing the initial distribution.

In separator imaging the problem is to measure the different interface levels inside the separator. The new algorithm is ideal for this application; the parameterization to use is obvious (*i.e.* different interface heights) and the number of ieeded parameters is relatively low. The latter makes it possible to pre-calculate all possible parameter combinations, and hence, a considerable decrease in reconstruction time results in comparison to the use of the finite element code for on-line capacitance calculations. For this application the different interface heights were measured within an accuracy of *1 cm*, and the time response (*i.e.* image rate) was approximately *1 second*.

Obtaining high quality reconstruction on the basis of limited number of capacitance data is a challenge, and scientists should be encouraged to develope reconstruction algorithm for different applications and speed demands.

6.   References

[1]   Huang S M, Xie C G, Thorn R, Snowden D, and Beck M S (1992) Design of sensor electronic for electrical capacitance tomography IEE Proceedings **Vol. 39** [1] 83-88.

[2]   Copley D C, Eberhard J W and Mohr G A (1994) Computed Tomography Part I: Introduction and Industrial Applications JOM January 1994

[3]   Xie C G, Huang S M, Hoyle B S, Thorn R, Lenn C, and Beck M S (1992) Electrical Capacitance Tomography for Flow Imaging - System model for development of reconstruction algorithms and design of primary sensors IEE Proceeding G **Vol. 139** No.1 (Febr. 1992) 89-98.

[4]   Isaksen Ø (1994) A Novel Approach to Reconstruction of Process Tomography Data PhD Thesis, University of Bergen, Norway

[5]   Isaksen Ø (1989) Imaging of two component pipe flow by use of capacitance sensors M.Sc. Thesis (in Norwegian) University of Bergen Norway.

[6]   Isaksen Ø and Nordtvedt J E (1993) A New Reconstruction Algorithm for Process Tomography Measurement, Science & Technology 1993, **Vol. 4**, No. 12, 1464-1475.

[7]   Isaksen Ø, Dico A S and Hammer E A (1994) A Capacitance based Tomography System for Interface Measurement in Separation Vessels Measurement, Science & Technology 1994, **Vol. 5**, No. 10., 1262-1271.

[8]   Isaksen Ø and Nordtvedt J E (1994) An Implicit Model based Reconstruction Algorithm for use with a Capacitance Tomography System Reviewed Proceedings of the third ECAPT conference (European Concerted Action on Process Tomography) Porto Portugal 24-26 March 1994.

[9]   Chen Q, Hoyle B S and Strangeways (1992) Electrical Field Interaction and an Enhanced Reconstruction Algorithm In Capacitance Process Tomography. Proceedings of the first ECAPT conference (European Concerted Action on Process Tomography) Manchester England 26-29 March 1994 ISBN: 1-85312-246-7 Southampton 205-212.

[10]   Nooralahiyan A Y, Hoyle B S and Bailey N J (1994) Application of a Neural Network in Imaging Reconstruction for Capacitance Tomography Reviewed Proceedings of the third ECAPT conference (European Concerted Action on Process Tomography) Porto Portugal 22-26 March 1994.

[11]   Reinecke N and Mewes D (1994) Resolution enhancement for multi-electrode capacitance sensors. Reviewed Proceedings of the third ECAPT conference (European Concerted Action on Process Tomography) Porto Portugal 22-26 March 1994.

[12]   Isaksen Ø and Nordtvedt J E (1992) Capacitance Tomography: Reconstruction Based on Optimization Theory Proceedings of the first ECAPT conference (European Concerted Activity on Process Tomography) Manchester England 26-29 March 1992 ISBN: 1-85312-246-7 Southampton 213-224.

[13]   Isaksen Ø and Nordtvedt J E (1992) A New Reconstruction Algorithm for Use with Capacitance-based Process Tomography Proceedings of the International Conference on Electronic Measurement & Instrumentation (ICEMI) Tianjin China 20-22 Oct. 1992 393-398. Modelling Identification & Control 1994 **Vol. 15**, No. 1.

[14]   Gill P E, Murray W, and Wright M H (1981) Practical Optimization (London: Academic Press).

[15]   Maxwell J.C. (1881) A Treatise on Electricity & Magnetism Calender Press Oxford.

[16]   Bruggeman D.A.G (1881) Berechnung Versciedener Physikalischer Konstanten von Heterogenen Substanzen Annalen der Physik 5 Folge Band 24.

Chapter 12

Noise Effects on Reconstructed Images in Electrical Impedance Tomography

J. Artola and J. Dell
Computer Systems Engineering Group
Department of Electronics, University of York
York YO1 5DD U.K.

1 Introduction

The performance of optimisation algorithms applied to Electrical Impedance Tomography (EIT) have been analyzed widely with simulated and noise free data [1,2]. In this paper three different Inverse Solvers (Marquardt Newton-Raphson, Smoothing Constraint and Singular Value Decomposition) are evaluated with noisy data and the corresponding reconstructed images are shown together with their rms Voltage Error (RMS) and Normalized Conductivity Error (NCE):

$$\text{RMS} = \frac{1}{N} \sqrt{\sum_{i=1}^{N} \left[\frac{(V_m)_i - (V_c)_i}{(V_c)_i} \right]^2} \qquad \text{NCE} = \frac{(\sigma - \sigma^k)^T (\sigma - \sigma^k)}{(\sigma - \sigma_a)^T (\sigma - \sigma_a)}$$

with

V_c = voltage set corresponding to the FEM model

V_m = measured voltage set

N = number of measurements

σ = original conductivity

σ^k = FEM conductivity vector in the kth iteration

σ_a = average of original conductivity.

In order to assess the influence of different noise levels in the measured data on the performance of these algorithms, a small percentage of noise (α) was added to the simulated voltage set (V) as follows:

$$V_i = V_i + \varepsilon_i \alpha V_i \qquad (1)$$

where ε_i represents a Gaussian random variable between 0 and 1.

Practice shows that both statistics are well behaved in the sense that when the normalized Conductivity Error between two given conductivity distributions is large, the corresponding rms Voltage Error is also large. Also rms Voltage Error is small for small values of normalized Conductivity Error. This is an indication that the rms Voltage Error can be used as an indication of whether a given algorithm is converging to the true conductivity or not.

This is no longer true when the measured voltages are contaminated with noise. This chapter shows how the algorithms that find the optimum conductivity distribution by minimising the rms Voltage Error alone fail when applied to noisy data. It is also shown that convergence can be improved by maximising the smoothness of the conductivity at the same time as minimising the rms Voltage Error.

2 Noise Effects in Reconstructed Images

The results presented in this chapter correspond to three different reconstruction algorithms based on optimisation techniques in which a given function (Φ) is minimised. This function depends on the difference between the measured voltage and the voltage calculated for a given conductivity distribution:

$$\Phi(\sigma) = \frac{1}{2}(J\Delta\sigma - \Delta V)^T(J\Delta\sigma - \Delta V) + \lambda\frac{1}{2}\Delta\sigma^T S\Delta\sigma \qquad (2)$$

Here ΔV represents the difference between the measured values and the voltages corresponding to the conductivity distribution calculated in the ith iteration. $\Delta\sigma$ is the conductivity update, and J is the Jacobian matrix whose elements are given by $J_{ij} = \frac{\partial v_i}{\partial \sigma_j}$.

Minimising this function means that the difference between measured and calculated voltages are minimised while also minimising some feature related to the conductivity update. This feature is reflected in the particular structure of the matrix S yet to be determined. The parameter λ indicates the relative importance of the two parts of the function Φ being minimised, i.e. for high levels of noise, λ will be considerably larger than one, so that the effects of the noise in the data is minimised.

The conductivity update is found by setting the derivative of the equation (2) equal to zero:

$$\frac{\partial \Phi(\Delta \sigma)}{\partial \Delta \sigma} = \mathbf{J}^T(\mathbf{J}\Delta\sigma - \Delta\mathbf{V}) + \lambda\,\mathbf{S}\Delta\sigma = 0$$

$$\Delta\sigma = (\mathbf{J}^T\mathbf{J} + \lambda\mathbf{S})^{-1}\mathbf{J}^T\Delta\mathbf{V}$$

Different types of regularisation techniques can be used, depending on the kind of *a priori* knowledge available, and this is reflected in the particular structure of the matrix S. Three different algorithms have been implemented in this research:

• In the special case when the conductivity oscillates near the initial guess the matrix S is the identity matrix. This regularisation technique, known as Marquardt's method [3], considerably improves the condition number of the Hessian matrix which has to be inverted, improving the stability of the algorithm as a result.

• When the conductivity is assumed to be smooth the S matrix is related to the smoothness of the conductivity update. Its effect is to minimise the rms Voltage Error while maximising the smoothness of the image [4,5].

• Singular Value Decomposition (SVD), in which the equation $\mathbf{J}\Delta\sigma=\Delta\mathbf{V}$ is solved. In this case the Jacobian matrix is decomposed into three matrices $\mathbf{U}^T\mathbf{W}\mathbf{V}$ [6] and some of the diagonal elements of the matrix W are set to zero before solving the system of equations [7].

In all three algorithms the conductivity values σ_i were constrained to be positive by applying the transformation [8]

$$\sigma_i = \exp(x_i) \qquad\qquad (3)$$

and minimising the difference between the calculated voltages and the measured voltages with respect to the new variables x_i. By using this transformation, the stability of the algorithm was improved and the peaks in the reconstructed image reduced.

These three algorithms are based on optimisation theory, in which a given value is minimised (in this case the difference between the measured voltage and the voltage corresponding to the theoretical model). Due to this feature, they are likely to be seriously affected by the presence of noise in the data.

In order to show the effect the added noise to the measurements has on the reconstructed images, the Forward Problem is solved for a particular (known) conductivity distribution and noise is added to the resulting voltages. The inverse problem is then solved and the reconstructed images and their statistics are shown.

Figure 1a shows the original phantom simulating a stratified flow. The dark zone has a conductivity of 4 mS/cm while the background conductivity is 2 mS/cm. The reconstructed images shown in (b)-(c) correspond to the Smoothing Constraint and Marquardt's Methods respectively. Ten percent Gaussian noise was added to the calculated voltages before solving the Inverse Problem. The graph (d) shows the rms Voltage Error for both methods corresponding to each iteration, and graph (e) shows the normalized Conductivity Error.

In a real case the original conductivity is unknown, so the normalized Conductivity Error can not be calculated. The only criterion available to assess convergence is the rms Error. If we are to trust the rms Error corresponding to Marquardt's method, Fig. 1d seems to suggest that the image after the third iteration is the most accurate or close to the original, since the algorithm converges (in the sense that the rms Error is smaller than in the previous iteration) during the first 3 iterations and then starts diverging.

Although practice shows that this criterion is generally acceptable for noise free data, it can no longer be applied when the measurements are contaminated with noise. Figure 1e supports this assessment. It can be seen that the normalized Conductivity

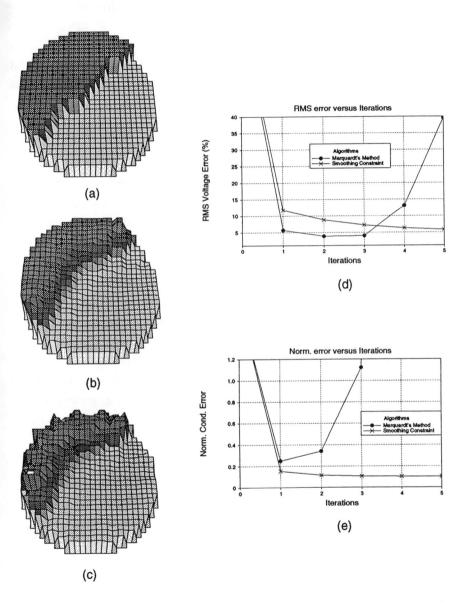

Figure 1: (a) Original Image. (b) and (c) Reconstructed images by using the Smoothing Constraint and Marquardt's Methods respectively. The rms error in (d) seems to indicate that the 3rd iteration is the most accurate for Marquardt's Method but the normalized error (e) shows that it is not the case.

Error increases after the first iteration of Marquardt's method, in clear contrast with the rms Error in Fig. 1d.

Both the rms and normalized Error in Fig. 1 (d)-(e) determined by the Smoothing Constraint method suggest that this method keeps converging even with further iterations. The improvement after the first iteration, however, is very small.

The results shown in Fig. 1 suggest that the decrease of the rms Error is no longer an indicator of convergence for Marquardt's method when the data is contaminated with noise. They also show that when the algorithm is applied to some of the phantoms, it starts diverging as early as the second iteration. This finding suggests that the algorithms must be stopped after the first iteration in order to get an image that can give some valuable information about the internal conductivity distribution. Further iterations are likely to degrade the image.

In Fig. 2 an original phantom (a) is used for solving the Forward Problem; the dark zones have a conductivity of 4 mS/cm and the background conductivity is 2 mS/cm. The resulting voltage set is degraded with both 10% and 20% noise levels, and the resulting reconstructed images-- corresponding to Marquardt's, Smoothing Constraint and SVD-- are shown after a single iteration. It can be seen that all of the methods give similar results and that no unexpected peaks are present in these reconstructions.

Given the initial conductivity distribution guess and the particular value of the parameter λ (or the number of diagonal elements to be set to zero in the case of the SVD algorithm) the inverse of the modified Hessian matrices (in the case of Marquardt and Smoothing Constraint algorithms) and the pseudoinverse (in the case of SVD algorithm) can be pre-calculated. This means that the computation per image is reduced to a matrix by a vector multiplication and some possibly some image processing routines, resulting in a fast reconstruction algorithm.

In order to explain why the first iteration converges while further iterations diverge, the Inverse Problem corresponding to a given original phantom is solved for noise free data. The graphs labeled "Iteration1-2" in Fig. 3 show the difference between the voltage at each electrode corresponding to the conductivity calculated in ith

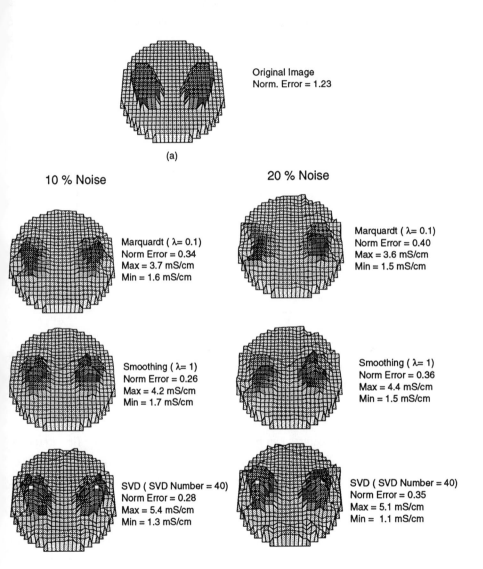

Figure 2: (a) Original Image. Reconstructed images for 10% added noise (left column) and 20% added noise (right column).

iteration and the voltages corresponding to the original phantom. The area between the x-axis and the line labeled "noise" shows where the noisy data would lie, if noise had been added according to equation (1). The graphs Iteration1-2 have been obtained however with noise free data.

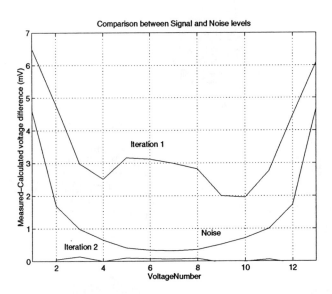

Fig. 3 The difference between the measured and the calculated voltages corresponding to the first two iterations are compared with the voltage corresponding to the original phantom. The maximum noise contribution is also shown.

Two important features can be seen in this graph: During the first iteration, graph "Iteration1", the maximum noise permitted is a small percentage (around 10%) of the difference between the two voltage sets near the centre (electrode 7), whereas the noise represents nearly 80% of the difference between the voltage sets near electrodes 1 & 13. Also, the graph corresponding to the second iteration is well below the maximum noise level (i.e. the noise is larger than the difference between two voltage sets), and the conductivity update calculated in this iteration is likely to be highly affected by the noise.

It can be seen that a second iteration is ineffective since the difference between the voltage sets is comparable with the noise. During the first iteration however, only

he data values near the the current drive electrodes (1, 2, 12, 13) are seriously affected
by noise, while for the rest the noise represents only a small percentage of the signal.
This can explain the success of some one-step iteration methods such as NOSER [9,
10] and Backprojection methods [11,12,13] in reconstructing images in the presence of
high levels of noise.

3 Artifacts due to the 2D assumption

The results shown in last sections are based on calculated data corresponding to
a 2 dimensional problem being applied to 2D Inverse solvers. In a real case, however,
the conductivity is 3 dimensional and this is likely to degrade the performance of these
algorithms. Ider [14] showed that when data corresponding to 3D object were directly
applied to 2D based reconstruction algorithms, the resulting image did not resemble the
original (using a backprojection method). In an attempt to solve this problem, he used
a normalization technique in which the 3D data is ``translated'' to 2D. This translation
is achieved by normalizing the measured data [1, 14]:

- The Forward Problem for the homogeneous case is solved in 2 and 3
dimensions, and the resulting voltages are stored in matrix $\mathbf{HV_2}$ and matrix $\mathbf{HV_3}$,
respectively.

- A correction vector β is calculated as

$$\beta_i = \frac{(\mathbf{HV_2})_i}{(\mathbf{HV_3})_i} \tag{4}$$

with i=1,2,...N, where N is the number of measurements.

- The measured 3D voltages ($\mathbf{V_3}$) corresponding to a non-homogeneous
conductivity are ``translated'' to the corresponding 2D version ($\mathbf{V_2}$) by using

$$(\mathbf{V_2})_i = \beta_i(\mathbf{V_3})_i \qquad i=1,2,...N. \tag{5}$$

Ider [14] showed that this simple adjustment improved the resulting image considerably when the algorithms were applied to 3D conductivity distribution independent of z.

This normalization procedure is tested by solving the Forward Problem for non-homogeneous conductivity in 3D, assuming that the conductivity is independent of the z coordinate. This assumption is valid when the system is applied to the measurement of conductivity profiles in human limbs (arms or legs), and it is certainly more correct than a 2D approximation. The 3D data are then normalized according to equations (4-5) and the resulting voltage is applied to the 2D Inverse Solvers. Figure 4 shows two original images together with their corresponding reconstructed images and statistics. Notice that these tests have been done with noise free data, so that the artifacts that can be seen in the reconstructed images are due to the 3D/2D voltage disparity. While the heterogeneities are clearly shown, their magnitude in the reconstructed images are 20% larger than in the original phantom, and some artifacts can be noted also.

4   Conclusions

It has been shown that the rms Voltage Error can no longer be used as an indication of convergence with Marquardt and SVD based algorithms when the data is contaminated with noise. Although the rms Voltage Error indicates that the algorithms are converging, they are really diverging in the sense that the normalized Conductivity Error increases after the first iteration. The Smoothing Constraint algorithm converges slowly (affecting both rms and NCE) and so, the rms Voltage Error can still be used in this case.

In order to assure a meaningful reconstructed image for every case, Marquardt and SVD methods must be stopped after the first iteration. Further iterations are likely to degrade the image, since the noise is comparable in magnitude with the signal. The Smoothing Constraint algorithm shows convergence with further iterations but this improvement is small in terms of NCE error.

It has been shown that the reconstructed image after the first iteration gives a good indication of the internal conductivity distribution, even with high levels of added Gaussian noise (up to 20%). It has also been shown that errors and artifacts are likely to appear in the reconstructed images when 2D algorithms are applied to data corresponding to 3D conductivity distributions. Consequently, a full 3D reconstruction algorithm is needed to avoid the artifacts due to the 2D approximations used so far.

References

1]   M. Z. Abdullah, Ph.D. thesis, University of Manchester, 1993.

2]   T. Y. Yorkey, J. G. Webster, and W. J. Tompkins, IEEE Transactions on Biomedical Engineering **34**:843-52 (1987).

[3]   D. W. Marquardt, J. Soc. Indust. Appl. Math. **11**:431-41, (1963).

[4]   E. L. Hall, Computer Image Processing and Recognition (Academic Press, New York, 1979).

[5]   P. Hua, E. J. Woo, J. G. Webster, and W. J. Tompkins, IEEE Trans. on Medical Imaging **10**:621-7 (1991).

[6]   G. H. Golub and C. F. Van Loan, Matrix Computations (Johns Hopkins University Press, Baltimore, 1989).

[7]   J. Artola, "A Study on Electrical Impedance Tomography (EIT) Reconstruction Algorithms", Ph.D. thesis, University of York, 1994.

[8]   Y. Sasaki, Memoirs of the Faculty of Engineering, Kyushu University **42**:59-74 (1982).

[9]   M. Cheney, D. Isaacson, J. C. Newell, S. Simske, and J. Goble J, Int. J. Imaging Systems and Technology **2**:66-75 (1990).

[10]   J. Goble, M. Cheney, and D. Isaacson, Appl. Computational Electromagnetic Society J. **7**:128-47 (1992).

[11]   D. C. Barber and B. H. Brown, Electronics Letters **19**:933-5, (1983).

[12]   C. J. Kotre, "Studies of Image Reconstruction Methods for Electrical Impedance Tomography", PhD thesis, Univ. Newcastle-upon-Tyne, 1993.

[13]   F. Santosa and M. Vogelius, SIAM J. Appl. Math **50**:216-43, (1990).

[14]   Y. Z. Ider and N. G. Gencer, IEEE Transactions on Medical Imaging **9**:49--59 (1990).

Chapter 13

Neural Networks for Image Reconstruction in Process Tomography

B. S. Hoyle, N. J. Bailey, A. Y. Nooralahiyan and D. M. Spink
Department of Electronic and Electrical Engineering
University of Leeds
Leeds, LS2 9JT, U.K.

Introduction

Many proposed process tomography (PT) methods are limited intrinsically by the computer processing needed for reconstruction; typically, powerful algorithms have a computer processing demand which is beyond the limits of real-time practicality for the dynamics of the target process. Some applications may require the use of supercomputers to obtain results in a reasonable amount of time.

Rapid progress in medical tomography in recent years presents the challenge of potential benefit to the industrial sector. Despite the temptation to consider such direct analogies, it is of course the case that the human body offers a simpler target: it is reasonably homogeneous, and for the most part its organs can be held in a stationary position during data capture. In the industrial case the target is likely to present large inhomogeneities and have intrinsic internal motion. Thus the challenge to the reconstruction processing task is severe: algorithms must cope with inhomogeneous targets and for many applications must be capable of fast evaluation.

Here we briefly review the use of parallel computing as a comparative means to deal with the processing demand and then explore what is perhaps the ultimate parallelism: the use of an artificial neural network (ANN) for the solution of the reconstruction problem. In general we concentrate upon PT systems in which sensors explore a field rather than track the path of a particle, so for example systems such as positron emission tomography (PET) are not considered.

2. Background

Many PT systems have successfully employed fast personal computers, relying upon the intrinsic processing capabilities of a particular microprocessor. When real-time performance has been critical, explicit parallel solutions have been used in which data parallelism is exploited in the acquisition process and algorithmic parallelism in the processing routines. This approach can lead to a scaleable solution in which the number of processors is matched to the particular speed requirements. Most applications have used the Inmos transputer as the processing element for these parallel systems [1, 2].

Much of the initial work on tomography was based on X-rays, for example the early description by Radon [3] of the concept of multiple projections. When the PT system is based upon an attenuation field (e.g. X-ray), the projection at an angle ϕ for the object function $f(x,y)$ was shown by Radon to be

$$\lambda(l,\phi) = \int_S f(x,y).ds \qquad (1)$$

The mapping defined by the projection along all possible lines of integration, S, is the (2-dimensional) *Radon transform* , *R* . A limited collection of projections, such as the multiple discrete application of eq. (1), is a *sample* of the Radon transform. If the projections are measured, as in a PT system, then an inverse transform may be used to estimate $f(x,y)$. The use of general purpose parallel computing systems for the forward and inverse evaluation of the Radon Transform has been explored, e.g. using transputers [5]. Systems have also been constructed from commercial digital signal processors [6] and specific purpose VLSI devices [7].

Most practical PT systems to date, in which measurement data is typically sparse, have taken a simple route to the general inversion problem based upon a *backprojection* algorithm. An analysis of the system is carried out to determine a set of data, or rules through which the multiple projection sensor data can be *back-*

projected to reveal information about the object function. The backprojections are typically overlaid, summed, and threshold filtered to yield an estimate of the function. Where possible *a priori* information can be used to remove reconstruction artefacts. The general concept of back-projection has seen many implementations: the use of sensitivity distributions in Electrical Capacitance Tomography (ECT) [2] and the use of circular and elliptical intersection arcs in ultrasonic reflection tomography [8].

For an ECT example backprojection yields a *greyscale* estimate of the permittivity object function distribution and may be summarised as

$$G(k_1) = c \sum_{i=1}^{m} \left\{ \mathbf{S}_j (k_1) \lambda_j \right\} \tag{2}$$

where m is the number of normalised capacitance measurements λ, c is the thresholding constant, and

$$\mathbf{S}_j = \frac{A}{A(k)} \frac{\mathbf{C}_j(k) - \mathbf{C}_j(\varepsilon_1)}{\mathbf{C}_j(\varepsilon_2) - \mathbf{C}_j(\varepsilon_1)} \frac{1}{\varepsilon_1 - \varepsilon_2} \tag{3}$$

defines the pre-computed sensitivity matrix. Here $A/A(k)$ is the ratio of the area of each k th element to the whole space, and $\mathbf{C}_{ij}(s)$ is the matrix of capacitance measurements between electrodes i and j for state, s . In (3) state s corresponds respectively to the space when full of material *1*, when full of material *2*, and when subjected to a small perturbation at k (of material *1* in the otherwise homogenous space containing *2*). S is typically computed using a finite element-based numerical field modeller which solves the *forward problem*. Eq. (1) depends upon the validity of S, which in turn implicitly assumes that the space contains only a small perturbation of material *1* in material *2*, e.g. gas in oil. *Soft field errors* will arise where this assumption is not justified, such as in mixtures containing materials of relatively high relative permittivity (e.g. water), or where there are large perturbations.

A number of trials have been made using ANNs to compute the inverse function through the association of measurement data with pre-taught patterns. Simple experimental trials using an ANN to reconstruct transmission mode ultrasound data aimed at medical systems were carried out by Conrath et al [9]. Further experimental trials of ANN's using ultrasound time of flight data have been carried out by Anthony et al [10] and Hutchins et al [11] for defect analysis. Morisue et al [12] have explored the use of a Hopfield ANN to computed tomography, based upon the algebraic reconstruction technique (ART). More applied trials have been carried out by Bidin et al [13] on the application of a Kohonen ANN for flow regime recognition in electrodynamic PT. Wetzler [14] has demonstrated the use of a multi-layer perceptron (MLP) ANN for pattern association in electrical impedance tomography (EIT) in solid-liquid flows. He uses a Sigma-Pi neuron model [15] due to its ability to incorporate non-linear characteristics, justified by the non-linear relationship between conductivity in the object space and node voltages in EIT.

3. A Single-Layer Multi-Output ANN

The authors have proposed a novel and simple ANN system addressed specifically at the association of PT measurement data and its interpretation. Trials have been carried out using ECT data for multi-component flow in an oil/gas/water pipeline [16-18]. The system consists of a primary network, which has the pattern association duty of estimating the cross sectional dielectric distribution, followed by a cascaded secondary network, whose task is the choice of flow regime from 4 candidates. Although the chosen example features ECT, the principles are considered to be applicable to other field-based PT systems. The primary network is trained with single element features, corresponding for example to a single gas bubble in an oil pipeline at each resolvable position. The secondary network is trained with idealised regimes for stratified, bubble, core and annular flow. The primary network is of key interest here due to its role in reconstruction.

3.1 Analysis of the SLMON

The primary network is a Single-Layer-Multi-Output-Network (SLMON) pattern associator. In the trials we used 54 neurons in the input layer (corresponding to the 66 capacitance measurements for a 12-electrode system, excluding the adjacent measurements) fully connected to a grid of 100 neurons in the output layer (corresponding to a 10x10 *pixel* spatial image), with no intra-layer connections. The secondary network is a MLP with one hidden layer trained with a back-propagation algorithm to identify four different flow regimes, namely: stratified, bubble, core and annular flow.

A single neuron defines a hyperplane of dimensions $(m-1)$, where m is the number of independent measurements made, in a m -dimensional Euclidean space which defines the pattern space [18-21]. For a single neuron to be capable of classifying a particular feature in pattern space, the region bounding the feature region must be clearly linearly separable by the hyperplane (called the decision plane) from all the other feature regions. Clearly the ECT problem is highly linearly separable: for a single neuron layer to classify 100 independent regions within the pipe from 54 independent measurements, 100 hyperplanes must be defined in a 54 dimension hyperspace. The fact that the problem is so high linearly separable is extraordinary and deserves investigation. The number of decision planes that can be put through N pattern regions in an n -dimension pattern space is given by the dichotomy of the problem $D(N,n)$:

$$D(N,n) = \begin{cases} 2\sum_{k=0}^{n}\left\{\dfrac{(N-1)!}{(N-1-k)!\,k!}\right\} & N > n \\ 2^{N} & N \le n \end{cases} \qquad (4)$$

The probability that a dichotomy chosen at random is a linearly separable decision function is

$$p(N,n) = \frac{D(N,n)}{2^{n}} \qquad (5)$$

As $N >> n$, the probability is very small. This degree of linear separability must mean that the feature regions in pattern space are highly organised, since each hyperplane must divide the feature space in such a way that the feature of interest lies on one side of the decision surface and all other features on the other side. In the special case of each element within the pipe only having the possibility of being in a high and low state, the pattern region is a point in pattern space.

Intuitively it is likely that patterns must lie on a continuously varying concave hypersurface, perhaps a hypersphere or hyperellipsoid. A study of the symmetries within our problem might give further indications about the shape of the surface. For instance, consider an element within a pipe that has 12 equally spaced electrodes. The pattern of the capacitance measurements, with this element in a high state, is the same as the pattern when the element is rotated about the centre of the pipe to any one of 11 other positions given by $(\theta + n360/12)$ degrees, but phase shifted by the rotation angle.

The hyperplane/decision function for a particular element in the space, k_1, is given by the equation

$$d(k_1) = \sum_{i=1}^{m-1} \sum_{j=i+1}^{m} \{w_j \lambda_j\} + w_{bias} \qquad (6)$$

When each pattern region is separable from the other regions by a single plane then (4) in vector form can be written

$$d(k_1) = \mathbf{w}^T \lambda_j \begin{cases} > 0 \Leftrightarrow \lambda_j \in \{k_1\} \\ \leq 0 \text{ otherwise} \end{cases} \qquad (7)$$

where $\mathbf{w}^T = \{w_{1,1}, w_{1,2}, w_{1,3}, \ldots, w_{m-1,m}\}$ is the set of "weights".

With neural networks a "squashing" function (usually a sigmoid function) is used after this step; although this function is used to derive the learning rule for training, it is not actually important for the functioning of a single layer of neurons. Therefore only function (7) will be used for generality. Important questions raised by this analysis are
- How can the weights be determined?
- What do they mean?
- Is there a link to the sensitivity analysis?

There is much literature on the determination of the weights of generalised decision functions; unfortunately almost all of the methods are iterative, apart from some very special cases. Although our problem does not fall into any of those special cases, it can be seen that if the feature regions lie on the hypersurface of something as simple as a hypersphere and their locations can be determined, this corresponds to a tangential hyperplane at that point. We need only to adjust the bias weight to translate the hyperplane into the correct position. The weights should also display the same rotational symmetry as the capacitance measurements. Indeed the weights found from iterative methods might give some indication of the shape.

Until now the training of the neurons has been with normalised capacitance values in which exactly one element's state is changed at a time. Some simple properties can be described about the size of weights:

1. If d is the decision function for element k_1, then

$$d(k_1) > 0$$
$$d(k_i) < 0 \ (k_i \in k_1')$$

and the weights must be such that $d(k_1) \geq -(d(k_2) + d(k_3) + ... + d(k_n))$.

2. The bias weight of all the neurons must be $w_{bias} < 0$ since when the pipe is empty, all of the elements are in a low state $d(k_i) < 0$.

3. The size of the weights should display the same rotational symmetry as the measured capacitance values.

3.2 SLMON Performance Analysis

Trials have indicated the viability of the approach described above. As outlined above the primary network is a SLMON with 54 neurons in the input layer (corresponding to a 12-electrode ECT system, excluding the adjacent measurements), fully connected to a grid of 100 neurons in the output layer (corresponding to the dielectric distribution). The secondary network is a MLP trained to identify stratified, bubble, core and annular flow regimes.

The performance of the composite system, outlined here, has been described in more detail elsewhere [22]. Results are presented as images, the finite element simulation (*phantom*) of each flow pattern is displayed on the left, with neural network images of gas/oil and water/oil to its right. Two thresholds are used to distinguish three components in the image. In the case of gas/oil flow these are: oil, gas/oil mixture (foam) and gas, for oil/water flow the component correspond to oil, oil/water mixture (emulsion) and water. The phantom displays the void fraction of gas (shown in white) in oil (light grey shaded area) within the cross section of the pipe. The water fraction in the image is shown in a darker shade, and the emulsion and the foam are outlined in both images. The references for both networks are displayed at the top of the image, for example, G_O_SIG_71gn refers to a trained gas/oil network with a 'sigmoid' thresholding function, and W_O_SIG_71wn refers to the corresponding water/oil network (see Fig 1). The output of SLMON is mapped to the cross section of the pipe, and the images indicate the firing of individual neurons correlating to the area of void fraction of the phantom. Fig 1 shows flow regime configurations for stratified and annular flow with void fractions of VOID_F = 0.262 and 0.48 respectively. SLMON maintains its fidelity (the accuracy of void fraction with respect to the simulated phantom) as well as relatively correct position of firing neurons.

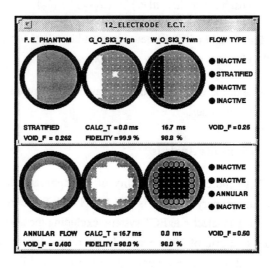

Fig. 1. - Stratified and Annular Flow Regimes

The reported calculation time is simply the workstation clock cycles, in these cases offering real-time performance of over 50 frames per second. Implementations could feasibly have much higher speeds.

3.3 The Effects of Noise on Performance

The data sets in trials were for two identical bubbles placed at the opposite edges of the pipe. The signal to noise ratio (S/N) is defined as signal power (averaged over all the input data set), divided by the power of gaussian noise, and it is reduced in stages, starting at 10dB, which produces almost perfect images. At about 5dB the reconstructed image for gas/oil network begins to degrade. Reducing S/N ratio to 1dB results in further degradation for the gas/oil network and much distortion in the image. The water/oil network on the other hand maintains its high accuracy and only begins to show deterioration at about -10dB. This effect can be understood by the relatively large permittivity difference in water/oil (about 80 to 3 respectively) compared to that of gas/oil (about 1 to 3 respectively). Tests for the smallest identifiable bubble in the centre of the pipe show that the water/oil image begins its deterioration at the lower level of about 3-4dB which is proposed as the noise limit for the water/oil reconstructor.

3.4 The Effect of Parameter Changes on Performance

In a set of trials the permittivity of the simulated water component was reduced in stages to determine the capability of SLMON to interpolate between the two components. The water/oil network is trained with component permittivities of 80 and 3 respectively. A linear thresholding function is used to allow the output to reflect the increase in permittivity as well as a reduction in permittivity of water. The tests carried out consists of water permittivity changes in the range of 20 to 200. Preliminary results indicate that SLMON consistently reflects the reduction in permittivity in the correct position.

The benefit of multi-layer networks with a non-linear thresholding function such as a sigmoid function is in the flexibility of representation and approximation of arbitrary functions. The output of a single layer network with linear thresholding function is simply the input vector (capacitance measurements) multiplied by the weight matrix (obtained after training).

3.5 Effects of Water and Oil Continuous Flows

A single network has been trained to reconstruct water continuous flow as well as oil continuous flow regimes. Examples presented are based upon training sets which consists mainly of the smallest identifiable element of high permittivity component (water droplets) placed in different positions within the low permittivity component (oil), and visa-versa, i.e. training one network for oil continuous and water continuous flows. The combined training sets cover the entire cross section of the pipe. Fig 2 illustrates the reconstructed image of a water droplet in oil as well as the oil droplet in water.

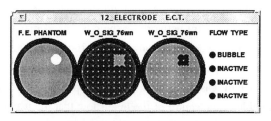

Fig. 2 - Water Continuous and Oil Continuous Flows

The significance of this network is its sensitivity to a small oil droplet in the position shown. Clearly a single high permittivity water droplet in otherwise low permittivity oil would have an appreciable effect on the measurement set; however the network can just as easily cope with a low permittivity oil droplet in an otherwise high permittivity water flow.

4. Conclusions

Proposals for the decision capabilities of the SLMON analysed above are demonstrated in the trials. A trained SLMON can make optimum use of variations in a measured data set and associate the extracted features from the input pattern, to that of training sets, to reconstruct images at high speed. SLMON can be trained to recognise two-component flows and produce comparable quality of output, regardless of the relative differences in component permittivities. This result alleviates the problem of distortion of the field (soft-field effect) and the consequential problems experienced in conventional image reconstruction algorithms. Thus a SLMON trained to identify say gas/oil flow is just as easily trained for oil/water flow without detriment to its performance.

The spatial resolution of the image for a given number of may be improved by adding more neurons to SLMON and training the net for smaller identifiable elements. The resolution will of course be limited by sensitivity of electrodes to detect capacitance changes.

SLMON has performed well with simulated noisy data sets, especially with large permittivity difference where individual measurements can be much larger than the average signal, thus enabling an easier feature detection process. Such noise performance is a particularly strong feature of the neural network approach in image reconstruction. SLMON can also reflect the permittivity changes; the output neurons with a linear thresholding function can extrapolate as well as interpolate to reflect permittivity variations of say water in oil.

We have shown that a single network can be trained to identify a small fraction of low permittivity component (oil) in water continuous flow, as well as a small fraction of high permittivity component (water) in oil continuous flow. This work illustrates the possibility of investigating links between the back-projection matrix of the conventional algorithm with the training weights of the SLMON.

5. References

[1]   F. Wiegand and B. S. Hoyle, Parallel Computing **17** 791-807 (1991).

[2]   C. G .Xie, S. M. Huang, B. S. Hoyle, R. Thorn, C. Lenn, D. Snowden and M.S.Beck, Proceedings IEE Part G **139** 89-98 (1992).

[3]   J. Radon, Ber. Sächische Akademie der Wissenschaften, **29**, 262-279 (1917).

[4]   G. Hall, T. J. Terrell, and L. M. Murphy, in Image processing and transputers, ed.H. C. Webber (IOS Press, Amsterdam, 1992), pp.47-72.

[5]   E. Shieh, W. Current, P. Hurst and I. Agi in Proceedings of IEEE 1990 Symposium on Circuits and Systems (IEEE, New York, 1990), pp234-237.

[6]   I. Agi, P. Hurst, W. Current, E. Shieh, S. Azevedo and G. Ford, Proc. SPIE **1246** 11-24 (1990).

[7]   S. J .Norton and M. Linzer, Ultrasonic Imaging **1** 154-184 (1979).

[8]   B. C. Conrath, C. M. W. Daft, W. D. O'Brien in Proceedings of IEEE 1989 Symposium on Ultrasonics (IEEE, New York, 1989), pp1007-1010.

[9] D. M. Anthony, E. L. Hines, D. A. Hutchins, and J. T. Mottram, Neural Computation **4** 758-771 (1992).

[10] D. A .Hutchins, J. T. Mottram, E. L. Hines, P. Corcoron and D. M. Anthony, in Proceedings of IEEE 1992 Symposium on Ultrasonics (IEEE, New York, 1992), pp365-368.

[11] M. Morisue, K. Sakai, and H. Koinuma, in Proceedings of IEEE 1992 Symposium on Circuits and Systems (IEEE, New York, 1992), pp2893-2896.

[12] A. R. Bidin, R. G. Green, M. E. Shackleton and R. W. Taylor, in Proceedings ECAPT '94, ed M.S.Beck et al. (UMIST, Manchester, 1994), pp203-214.

[13] D. Wetzler, Proceedings ECAPT '94, ed. M.S.Beck et al. (UMIST, Manchester, 1994), pp276-284.

[14] H. C. Yau, M.T.Mantry, Neural networks, **3** 437-443 (1990).

[15] A. Y. Nooralahiyan, B. S. Hoyle, N. J. Bailey, in Proceedings ECAPT '93, ed M.S.Beck et al. (UMIST, Manchester, 1994), pp50-53.

[16] A. Y. Nooralahiyan, B. S. Hoyle, N. J. Bailey, in Proceedings ECAPT '94, ed M.S.Beck et al. (UMIST, Manchester, 1994), pp266-276.

[17] A. Y. Nooralahiyan, B. S. Hoyle, and N. J. Bailey, Proceeding IEE Circuits, Devices and Systems, **141** 517-521 (1994).

[18] R P. Lippmann, IEEE ASSP Magazine, **3** pp4-22 (1987).

[19] L. McClelland and D. Rumelhart, Exploration in Parallel Distributed Processing, (The MIT Press, 1991).

[20] R. Beale, T. Jackson, Neural Computing an Introduction, (Adam Hilger, 1991).

[21] J. M. Zurada, Introduction to Artificial Neural Systems, (West, 1992).

[22] A. Y. Nooralahiyan, B. S. Hoyle, N. J. Bailey, in Proceedings ECAPT '95, ed M.S.Beck et al. (UMIST, Manchester, 1995), pp420-424.

Chapter 14

Direct Algebraic Reconstruction in Electromagnetic Flow Tomography

A. Trächtler, A. Wernsdörfer,
Institut für Meß- und Regelungstechnik,
Universität (T.H.) Karlsruhe
Postfach 6980, D–76128 Karlsruhe, Germany

1. Introduction

Electromagnetic flow measurement has asserted many fields of application due to its non-invasive measuring principle and accuracy. The conventional set-up is depicted in Fig. 1 a. An externally excited magnetic field $\vec{B}$ penetrates a pipe perpendicular to the flow velocity $v_z(\vec{x})$ of a conductive fluid inducing an electric field. The resulting voltage is measured between two electrodes aligned perpendicular to both the magnetic field and the flow velocity and yields a value being proportional to the mean flow velocity, provided that the flow profile is axially symmetric. Otherwise, the flowmeter gives erroneous results. This systematic error due to flow profile can be reduced using more than one pair of electrodes and various magnetic fields [1], [2] (cf. Fig. 1 b).

In this contribution, not measurement of the mean flow velocity, but tomographic reconstruction of the flow profile is investigated based on the scheme of Fig. 1 b. Flow profile reconstruction was already proposed in [3] using series expansion methods with Fourier-Bessel or discrete pixel basis-functions. Here, we give the analytical foundations of electromagnetic flow tomography, prove the uniqueness of the inverse problem, and derive an analytical reconstruction procedure (second

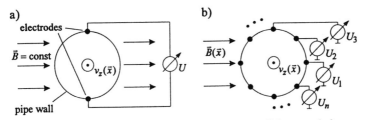

Fig. 1: Electromagnetic flow measurement. Scheme of the conventional (a), and enhanced (b) set-up.

section). In the third section, we apply the *Direct-Algebraic-Reconstruction* method (DAR), known from image reconstruction [4], [5], to electromagnetic flow tomography, and in the fourth section the good performance of DAR is demonstrated by simulation.

Under the aspect of mathematical modelling the measurement, the various tomographic reconstruction methods can be classified into three groups: analytical, direct algebraic, and discrete reconstruction methods, respectively (Table 1).

In analytical methods (e.g. Direct Fourier Method, Filtered Backprojection, Radon's inversion formula [6]) the measured data are assumed to be an infinite, continuous set allowing theoretically an exact inversion. In practice, only a discrete, finite set of measurements is available, thus infinitesimal operations as integration and differentiation have to be approximated by sums and differences. Obviously, if the amount of data is small, these approximations are bad, and the resulting reconstruction is not satisfying.

In contrast, the discrete methods (as ART, its variations, and series expansion methods) deal with the discrete measurements, and the continuous field is approximated by a discrete set of data (pixels, or coefficients of truncated series). This model leads to a set of linear equations, which must be solved for reconstruction (by pseudo-inversion). Here, the measurement is modelled inadequately, and the spatial resolution of the reconstructed image may be too low.

With Direct Algebraic Reconstruction the disadvantages of the above mentioned methods are avoided. According to physical reality, in DAR the measurement is considered as a mapping from the continuous 2D-field (an element of a function space) onto the vector of measured data (element of a finite-dimensional vector space). Optimal reconstruction means pseudo-inversion of this mapping, where the pseudo-inverse operator is a mapping from the vector space onto the function space. Thus, an arbitrary spatial resolution can be achieved, and no errors are made in modelling measurement.

Table 1: Classification of tomographic reconstruction methods

reconstruction:		analytic	direct algebraic	discrete
measurement:	field	continuous	continuous	discrete
map of the field	↓	↓	↓	↓
onto the data	data	continuous	discrete	discrete

2. Theory of electromagnetic flow tomography

Electromagnetic flow measurement is based on Lorentz' force inducing an electric field

$$\vec{E}(\vec{x}) = \vec{v}(\vec{x}) \times \vec{B}(\vec{x}) \tag{1}$$

in a conductive fluid, where $\vec{v}(\vec{x})$ denotes the fluid velocity field, and $\vec{B}(\vec{x})$ the magnetic induction.

The measured quantity is the resulting potential distribution $U(\vec{x})$ at the pipe wall, which is generally given by [7], [8]:

$$U(\vec{x}) = \iiint \vec{v}(\vec{x}') \cdot \left[\mathrm{grad}'G(\vec{x}, \vec{x}') \times \vec{B}(\vec{x}')\right] \mathrm{d}^3 x'. \tag{2}$$

Herein, $G(\vec{x}, \vec{x}')$ denotes the Green's function of the pipe with Neumann's boundary conditions. For simplicity, the pipe is considered to have an infinite length; the pipe axis coincides with the z-axis, and the pipe radius is normalized to unity. Additionally, it is assumed that all quantities are independent of z, and that the velocity field has only the single component v_z in z-direction. Then the voltage at the pipe wall is given by a surface integral over the cross section Ω of the pipe:

$$U(\vec{x}) = \iint_\Omega v_z \left(\frac{\partial G}{\partial x'} B_y - \frac{\partial G}{\partial y'} B_x\right) \mathrm{d}^2 x', \quad \Omega: \text{unit circle.} \tag{3}$$

Here, $G(\vec{x}, \vec{x}')$ is the Green's function of the unit circle (with Neumann's boundary conditions).

Using polar coordinates for both the position of the electrodes $\vec{x} = [\cos\varphi, \sin\varphi]$ at the pipe wall and the integration variables $\vec{x}' = r'[\cos\varphi', \sin\varphi']$ in the pipe, the Green's function $G(\vec{x}, \vec{x}')$ is given by [9]

$$G(\vec{x}, \vec{x}') = -\frac{1}{2\pi}\ln\left(1 - 2r'\cos(\varphi' - \varphi) + r'^2\right) = \tag{4}$$

$$= \frac{1}{\pi}\sum_{k=1}^\infty \frac{1}{k} r'^k \cos k(\varphi' - \varphi), \quad 0 \le \varphi', \varphi < 2\pi; \quad 0 \le r' < 1. \tag{5}$$

Whereas the magnetic fields used practically are as simple as possible (e.g. fields which are constant or have constant first and higher gradients within the pipe), for theoretical analysis other fields are applied. Since the exciting coils are outside the pipe, the magnetic field inside the pipe is source- and curl-free thus being the curl of a harmonic vector potential:

$$\vec{B} = -\mathrm{curl}\vec{A}, \quad \text{in two dimensions:} \quad \vec{B} = \begin{bmatrix} B_x \\ B_y \end{bmatrix} = \begin{bmatrix} -\partial A/\partial y \\ \partial A/\partial x \end{bmatrix}. \tag{6}$$

The functions being harmonic in the unit circle are $r^n \cos n\varphi$, $r^n \sin n\varphi$, $n = 1, 2, \ldots$ and linear combinations. We choose

$$A_n = \frac{r^{n+1}}{n+1}\cos(n+1)\varphi, \quad \vec{B}_n = -\mathrm{curl}A_n = r^n \begin{bmatrix} \sin n\varphi \\ \cos n\varphi \end{bmatrix}, \quad n = 0, 1, 2, \ldots \tag{7}$$

(It can be shown that the magnetic fields derived from the vector potentials $r^n \sin n\varphi$ yield exactly the same information; thus it is sufficient considering the fields in eq. (7)). The potential distribution resulting from the magnetic field $\vec{B}_n$ is denoted by U_n; U_n is a function of the azimuth angle of the electrode position at the pipe wall:

$$U_n(\varphi) = \int\limits_{r'=0}^{1} \int\limits_{\varphi'=0}^{2\pi} v_z \left(\frac{\partial G}{\partial x'} B_{n,y} - \frac{\partial G}{\partial y'} B_{n,x} \right) r' d\varphi' dr' . \tag{8}$$

The velocity field $v_z(x,y)$ is expanded into a Fourier series with respect to the angle φ:

$$v_z(x,y) = \frac{1}{2} c_0(r) + \sum_{k=1}^{\infty} c_k(r) \cos k\varphi + d_k(r) \sin k\varphi , \quad \text{where} \tag{9}$$

$$\begin{bmatrix} c_k(r) \\ d_k(r) \end{bmatrix} = \frac{1}{\pi} \int_0^{2\pi} v_z(r \cos \varphi, r \sin \varphi) \begin{bmatrix} \cos k\varphi \\ \sin k\varphi \end{bmatrix} d\varphi , \quad k = (0,)1,2,\ldots . \tag{10}$$

Inserting (9), (7), and (5) into (8) and integrating over φ' , finally results in

$$U_n(\varphi) = M_{2n+1}\{c_0(r)\}\cos(n+1)\varphi +$$
$$+ \sum_{k=1}^{\infty} M_{2n+k+1}\{c_k(r)\}\cos(n+k+1)\varphi + M_{2n+k+1}\{d_k(r)\} \sin(n+k+1)\varphi +$$
$$+ \sum_{k=1}^{n} M_{2n-k+1}\{c_k(r)\}\cos(n-k+1)\varphi - M_{2n-k+1}\{d_k(r)\} \sin(n-k+1)\varphi .$$
$$\tag{11}$$

Herein,

$$M_\nu\{c_k(r)\} = \int\limits_{r=0}^{\infty} c_k(r)r^\nu dr , \quad M_\nu\{d_k(r)\} = \int\limits_{r=0}^{\infty} d_k(r)r^\nu dr , \quad \nu = 0,1,2,\ldots \tag{12}$$

are the ν-th order moments of the coefficient functions $c_k(r)$ and $d_k(r)$.

On the basis of eq. (11) the information over $v_z(x,y)$ obtained by measuring the potential distributions $U_n(\varphi)$ can be interpretated: Expanding $U_n(\varphi)$ into a Fourier-series, the corresponding Fourier coefficients are, according to the first and second line of eq. (11), given by the moments

$$M_{2n+k+1}\{c_k(r)\} , \quad M_{2n+k+1}\{d_k(r)\} , \quad k = (0,)1,2,\ldots \quad n = 0,1,2,\ldots \tag{13}$$

of the coefficient functions $c_k(r)$, $d_k(r)$ from the Fourier series (9) of the velocity field $v_z(x,y)$ searched for. (The moments occuring in the third line of eq. (11) are contained in (13), too, with suitably changed indices.)

The remaining question is, whether the knowledge of the moments (13) is sufficient for reconstructing $v_z(x,y)$, and how to get a reconstruction procedure. This can be worked out in the frequency domain of Fourier transform.

The two-dimensional Fourier transform of $v_z(x,y)$,

$$V_z(\omega_x,\omega_y) = \int\limits_{-\infty}^{\infty} \int\limits_{-\infty}^{\infty} v_z(x,y)e^{-j(\omega_x x+\omega_y y)}\,dxdy\,, \qquad (14)$$

using polar coordinates

$$\omega_x = \omega_r \cos\psi\,, \quad \omega_y = \omega_r \sin\psi \qquad (15)$$

and the series expansion (9), is given by

$$V_z(\omega_x,\omega_y) = 2\pi \left\{ \frac{1}{2}C_0(\omega_r) + \sum_{k=1}^{\infty}(-j)^k \Big(C_k(\omega_r)\cos k\psi + D_k(\omega_r)\sin k\psi \Big) \right\}\,. \qquad (16)$$

Here, the coefficient functions $C_k(\omega_r)$, $D_k(\omega_r)$ are the k-th order Hankel transforms of $c_k(r)$ and $d_k(r)$, respectively [10]:

$$\left[\begin{array}{c} C_k(\omega_r) \\ D_k(\omega_r) \end{array}\right] = \int\limits_0^{\infty} r \left[\begin{array}{c} c_k(r) \\ d_k(r) \end{array}\right] J_k(\omega_r r)\,dr,\ k = (0,)1,2,\dots\,. \qquad (17)$$

$J_k(x)$ is the k-th order Bessel function. Expanding the Hankel transforms $C_k(\omega_r)$, $D_k(\omega_r)$ into power series about $\omega_r = 0$, yields

$$\begin{aligned} C_k(\omega_r) &= \sum_{n=0}^{\infty} \frac{(-1)^n}{n!(n+k)!}M_{2n+k+1}\{c_k(r)\}\left(\frac{\omega_r}{2}\right)^{2n+k}\,, \\ D_k(\omega_r) &= \sum_{n=0}^{\infty} \frac{(-1)^n}{n!(n+k)!}M_{2n+k+1}\{d_k(r)\}\left(\frac{\omega_r}{2}\right)^{2n+k}\,. \end{aligned} \qquad (18)$$

This is the so-called moment theorem of the Hankel transform [10]. In the power series (18) just those moments (13) occur which are known from voltage measurement. It can be shown that the radius of convergence of the power series is ∞. Thus it is possible to calculate the functions $C_k(\omega_r)$, $D_k(\omega_r)$ and then the spectrum $V_z(\omega_x,\omega_y)$ from the moments $M_{2n+k+1}\{c_k(r)\}$, $M_{2n+k+1}\{d_k(r)\}$ which are known by measurement. Finally, one obtains the velocity field $v_z(x,y)$ searched for by two-dimensional inverse Fourier transform. A scheme of this reconstruction procedure is depicted in Fig. 2. We point to the parallelism to the Central Slice

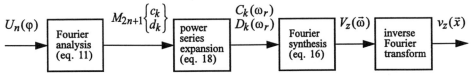

Fig. 2: Scheme of the analytical reconstruction procedure
in electromagnetic flow tomography.

Theorem and to the Direct Fourier Method of conventional tomography [6]. So far, the theoretical part dealing with uniqueness of reconstruction, measurement data needed for complete reconstruction, and analytic reconstruction procedure is completed.

3. Tomographic reconstruction with DAR

The relation between the measured data and the distribution of the measurand in the frequency domain presented in the previous section is one possible approach of a direct reconstruction comparable to the Direct Fourier method in conventional tomography [6]. However, its results are not always satisfying, particularly if the amount of data is small, and therefore it is used rarely. For the performance of other approaches it is very important that their mathematical models express the reality as good as possible. With the DAR the physical conditions given by the particular problem can be covered very well. Additionally, in contrast to other methods no improper assumptions concerning the structure of the data or of the function searched for must be made, e.g. a discretization of the investigated area is not needed.

For the DAR the measurement is considered as a mapping of elements of one Hilbert space to another one. Usually, the $L_\varrho^2(\Omega)$, the space of ϱ-square-integrable functions over the domain Ω (ϱ: weighting function; Ω is in our context the unit circle), is used as space for the function searched for, and for the data, due to their discrete nature, the finite dimensional space $\mathbb{R}^m$ of vectors with m real elements is used. $m = K \cdot N$ is the total number of measurements, where in this case N denotes the number of different magnetic fields and K the number of electrodes (in Fig. 1 b: $K = 8$). The integral representing a single tomographic measurement is considered as an inner product $\langle \cdot, \cdot \rangle_{L_\varrho^2(\Omega)}$

$$u_i = \langle \kappa_i(\vec{x}), v_z(\vec{x}) \rangle_{L_\varrho^2(\Omega)} \tag{19}$$

of the investigated function $v_z(\vec{x})$ and a characteristic function $\kappa_i(\vec{x})$. $\kappa_i(\vec{x})$ permits a precise modelling of the physics of the measurement. For electromagnetic flow measurement eq. (8) for the i-th measurement with magnetic field $\vec{B}_{n_i}$ and position of the electrodes $\vec{x}_{k_i} = [\cos\varphi_{k_i}, \sin\varphi_{k_i}]$ becomes

$$
\begin{aligned}
u_i &= U_{n_i}(\varphi_{k_i}) = \iint_\Omega v_z(\vec{x}') \left(\frac{\partial G(\vec{x}_{k_i}, \vec{x}')}{\partial x'} B_{n_i,y} - \frac{\partial G(\vec{x}_{k_i}, \vec{x}')}{\partial y'} B_{n_i,x} \right) \mathrm{d}^2 x' = \\
&= \iint_\Omega \underbrace{\frac{1}{(1-r'^2)^2}}_{\varrho(\vec{x}')} \underbrace{(1-r'^2)^2 \left(\frac{\partial G(\vec{x}_{k_i}, \vec{x}')}{\partial x'} B_{n_i,y} - \frac{\partial G(\vec{x}_{k_i}, \vec{x}')}{\partial y'} B_{n_i,x} \right)}_{\kappa_i(\vec{x}')} v_z(\vec{x}') \, \mathrm{d}^2 x' = \\
&= \iint_\Omega \varrho(\vec{x}') \, \kappa_i(\vec{x}') \, v_z(\vec{x}') \, \mathrm{d}^2 x' = \langle \kappa_i(\vec{x}), v_z(\vec{x}) \rangle_{L_\varrho^2(\Omega)} = W_i \, v_z(\vec{x}).
\end{aligned}
\tag{20}
$$

The weighting function $\varrho(\vec{x})$ was suitably chosen, so that $\kappa_i(\vec{x}') \in L_\varrho^2(\Omega)$. With the Green's function and the magnetic fields from eqs. (4,7), the characteristic function κ_i becomes

$$\kappa_i(\vec{x}) = \frac{1}{\pi}(1-r)^2 \, r^{n_i} \, \frac{\cos(n_i \varphi + \varphi_{k_i}) - r\cos(n_i + 1)\varphi}{1 - 2r\cos(\varphi - \varphi_{k_i}) + r^2} \, . \qquad (21)$$

The total of all measurements leads to the data vector

$$\vec{u} = \begin{bmatrix} u_1 \\ \vdots \\ u_m \end{bmatrix} = \begin{bmatrix} \langle \kappa_1(\vec{x}), v_z(\vec{x}) \rangle_{L^2_\varrho} \\ \vdots \\ \langle \kappa_m(\vec{x}), v_z(\vec{x}) \rangle_{L^2_\varrho} \end{bmatrix} = \begin{bmatrix} \mathcal{W}_1 v_z(\vec{x}) \\ \vdots \\ \mathcal{W}_m v_z(\vec{x}) \end{bmatrix} = \mathcal{W} v_z(\vec{x}) \, . \qquad (22)$$

Herein, $\mathcal{W}$ denotes the mapping operator $\mathcal{W} : L^2_\varrho(\Omega) \to \mathbb{R}^m$. If the inverse operator $\mathcal{W}^{-1}$ existed, the tomographic problem calculating $v_z(\vec{x})$ given $\vec{u}$ could be solved by applying $\mathcal{W}^{-1}$ to $\vec{u}$. Instead an optimal approximation $\hat{v}_z(\vec{x})$ is obtained by the pseudo-inverse operator $\mathcal{W}^+$

$$\hat{v}_z(\vec{x}) = \mathcal{W}^+ \vec{u} = \mathcal{W}^*(\mathcal{W}\mathcal{W}^*)^{-1}\vec{u} \, . \qquad (23)$$

$\mathcal{W}^*$ is the adjoint to $\mathcal{W}$ with $\mathcal{W}^* : \mathbb{R}^m \to L^2_\varrho(\Omega)$. This solution is optimal in the sense that it minimizes the norm of the residual $\|\vec{u} - \mathcal{W}\hat{v}_z(\vec{x})\|_{\mathbb{R}^m} \to \min$ and the norm $\|\hat{v}_z(\vec{x})\|_{L^2_\varrho} \to \min$. (The norm of an element a of a Hilbert space is defined by $\|a\| = \sqrt{\langle a, a \rangle}$.) In order to exploit eq. (23) a definition of $\mathcal{W}^*$ and a discussion of the operator $(\mathcal{W}\mathcal{W}^*)$ and its inversion is necessary.

The adjoint of a mapping operator between two Hilbert spaces is defined by the equivalence of the inner products in the two spaces:

$$\langle \vec{u}, \mathcal{W} v_z(\vec{x}) \rangle_{\mathbb{R}^m} \stackrel{\text{def.!}}{=} \langle \mathcal{W}^* \vec{u}, v_z(\vec{x}) \rangle_{L^2_\varrho(\Omega)} \, . \qquad (24)$$

The inner product in $\mathbb{R}^m$ is given by

$$\langle \vec{u}_1, \vec{u}_2 \rangle_{\mathbb{R}^m} = \sum_{i=1}^{m} u_{1_i} u_{2_i} \, . \qquad (25)$$

Together with eqs. (19) and (20), this yields

$$\langle \vec{u}, \mathcal{W} v_z(\vec{x}) \rangle_{\mathbb{R}^m} = \sum_{i=1}^{m} u_i \, \mathcal{W}_i v_z(\vec{x}) = \sum_{i=1}^{m} u_i \iint_\Omega \varrho(\vec{x}') \, \kappa_i(\vec{x}') \, v_z(\vec{x}') \, \mathrm{d}^2 x' =$$

$$= \iint_\Omega \varrho(\vec{x}') \left(\sum_{i=1}^{m} \kappa_i(\vec{x}') u_i \right) v_z(\vec{x}') \, \mathrm{d}^2 x' = \Big\langle \underbrace{\sum_{i=1}^{m} \kappa_i(\vec{x}) u_i}_{\mathcal{W}^* \vec{u}}, v_z(\vec{x}) \Big\rangle_{L^2_\varrho(\Omega)} =$$

$$= \langle \mathcal{W}^* \vec{u}, v_z(\vec{x}) \rangle_{L^2_\varrho(\Omega)} \, .$$

Thus, the adjoint $\mathcal{W}^*$ is given by

$$\mathcal{W}^* \vec{u} = \sum_{i=1}^{m} \kappa_i(\vec{x}) u_i \, , \qquad (26)$$

and is, applied to a vector $\vec{u} \in \mathbb{R}^m$, the superposition of the u_i weighted with the corresponding characteristic functions $\kappa_i(\vec{x})$.

Now the composite operator $\mathcal{W}\mathcal{W}^*$ is considered. $\mathcal{W}^*$ applied to a vector yields a function, and $\mathcal{W}$ applied to this function yields again a vector. Thus, $\mathcal{W}\mathcal{W}^*$ is a real $m \times m$ matrix, denoted by $\mathbf{W}$: $\mathbf{W} = \mathcal{W}\mathcal{W}^*$, which must be inverted in eq. (23). We denote the product of $\mathbf{W}^{-1}$ and $\vec{u}$ in eq. (23) with $\vec{\tilde{u}}$:

$$\vec{\tilde{u}} = \mathbf{W}^{-1}\vec{u} = (\mathcal{W}\mathcal{W}^*)^{-1}\vec{u}. \tag{27}$$

In order to get an instruction for the computation of the elements w_{ij} of $\mathbf{W}$ we consider the i-th equation of the linear set of equations $\vec{u} = \mathbf{W}\vec{\tilde{u}} = (\mathcal{W}\mathcal{W}^*)\vec{\tilde{u}}$:

$$
\begin{aligned}
u_i &= \mathcal{W}_i(\mathcal{W}^*\vec{\tilde{u}}) = \mathcal{W}_i \sum_{j=1}^m \kappa_j(\vec{x})\,\tilde{u}_j = \iint_\Omega \varrho(\vec{x}')\,\kappa_i(\vec{x}')\left(\sum_{j=1}^m \kappa_j(\vec{x}')\tilde{u}_j\right) \mathrm{d}^2 x' = \\
&= \sum_{j=1}^m \underbrace{\iint_\Omega \varrho(\vec{x}')\,\kappa_i(\vec{x}')\kappa_j(\vec{x}')\mathrm{d}^2 x'}_{w_{ij}}\,\tilde{u}_j = \sum_{j=1}^m w_{ij}\tilde{u}_j
\end{aligned}
$$

resulting to

$$w_{ij} = \iint_\Omega \varrho(\vec{x}')\,\kappa_i(\vec{x}')\kappa_j(\vec{x}')\mathrm{d}^2 x' = \langle \kappa_i(\vec{x}), \kappa_j(\vec{x})\rangle_{L^2_\varrho(\Omega)}. \tag{28}$$

A matrix element represents a surface integral of the characteristic functions $\kappa_i \cdot \kappa_j$ over Ω weighted with $\varrho(\vec{x})$, and hence is determined only by the measurement geometry and is the same for all data vectors of this set-up. Eq. (28) can be evaluated by numeric integration, but we calculated w_{ij} analytically by inserting the characteristic function κ_i from eq. (20) into eq. (28) and using the Green's function G and the magnetic fields $\vec{B}_n$ from the previous section. Omitting trigonometric acrobatics, the final result for the matrix element w_{ij} is:

$$w_{ij} = \frac{1}{2\pi}\left(H_1 + H_2\right), \qquad \text{with} \tag{29}$$

$$H_1 = \frac{1}{2(n_i + n_j + 1)(n_i + n_j + \frac{3}{2})(n_i + n_j + 2)} \sum_{\nu=1}^{n_i+n_j+1} \cos\left[\nu\beta_{ij} + (n_i + n_j + 2)\varphi_{k_j}\right],$$

and, if $\varphi_{k_i} = \varphi_{k_j}$:

$$H_2 = \cos(n_i - n_j)\varphi_{k_i}\left\{\frac{1}{2(n_i + 1)(n_i + \frac{3}{2})} - 4\ln 2 + 2 + 2\sum_{\nu=1}^{n_i+1}\frac{1}{\nu(4\nu^2 - 1)}\right\},$$

if $\varphi_{k_i} \neq \varphi_{k_j}$:

$$H_2 = -\left[\cos\gamma_{ij} + \cos(\gamma_{ij} + \beta_{ij})\right]\cdot\left[\ln\left(2\sin\frac{\beta_{ij}}{2}\right) + \sum_{\nu=1}^{n_i}\frac{\cos\nu\beta_{ij}}{\nu}\right] +$$

$$+\left[\sin\gamma_{ij}+\sin(\gamma_{ij}+\beta_{ij})\right]\cdot\left[\frac{\pi-\beta_{ij}}{2}-\sum_{\nu=1}^{n_i}\frac{\sin\nu\beta_{ij}}{\nu}\right]-\frac{\cos(n_i\beta_{ij}-\gamma_{ij})}{n_i+1}+$$

$$+4\sum_{\nu=0}^{n_i}\frac{\cos(\nu\beta_{ij}-\gamma_{ij})}{2\nu+1}+2\cos\left(\gamma_{ij}+\frac{\beta_{ij}}{2}\right)\cdot\ln\left(\tan\frac{\beta_{ij}}{4}\right)-\pi\sin\left(\gamma_{ij}+\frac{\beta_{ij}}{2}\right).$$

Herein, $\gamma_{ij}=n_j\varphi_{k_i}-n_i\varphi_{k_j}$, and $\beta_{ij}=\varphi_{k_i}-\varphi_{k_j}-2\nu\pi$ for $2\nu\pi\leq\varphi_{k_i}-\varphi_{k_j}<2(\nu+1)\pi$, $\nu=0,\pm1,\pm2,\ldots$ (i.e. $0\leq\beta_{ij}<2\pi$). The numerical costs for computing these matrix elements are of no importance because the matrix must be calculated only one time for a fixed measurement geometry, i.e. experimental set-up.

Finally, the reconstruction with DAR can be summarized as follows:

1. Calculate a new vector $\vec{\tilde{u}}$ given the measured data vector $\vec{u}$ by solving the linear set of equations $\mathbf{W}\vec{\tilde{u}}=(\mathcal{W}\mathcal{W}^*)\vec{\tilde{u}}=\vec{u}$:

$$\vec{\tilde{u}}=\mathbf{W}^{-1}\vec{u}=(\mathcal{W}\mathcal{W}^*)^{-1}\vec{u}.\tag{30}$$

Since the matrix $\mathbf{W}=\mathcal{W}\mathcal{W}^*$ can be ill-conditioned or even singular, regularizing methods like a truncated singular value decomposition must be used for the inversion.

2. Reconstruct $\hat{v}_z(\vec{x})$ at each desired position $\vec{x}\in\Omega$ by applying the adjoint mapping operator $\mathcal{W}^*$ to the new vector $\vec{\tilde{u}}$ according to eq. (23):

$$\hat{v}_z(\vec{x})=\mathcal{W}^*\vec{\tilde{u}}=\sum_{i=1}^{m}\kappa_i(\vec{x})\tilde{u}_i.\tag{31}$$

In the following section we will demonstrate the good performance of DAR with some simulations.

4. Simulations

For proving the advantages of DAR in the case of few data, we consider an enhanced electromagnetic flowmeter consisting of eight electrodes as depicted in Fig. 1 b (and one common ground electrode). According to eq. (7) we apply three magnetic fields:

$$\vec{B}_0=\begin{bmatrix}0\\1\end{bmatrix},\quad\vec{B}_1=r\begin{bmatrix}\sin\varphi\\\cos\varphi\end{bmatrix}=\begin{bmatrix}y\\x\end{bmatrix},\quad\vec{B}_2=r^2\begin{bmatrix}\sin 2\varphi\\\cos 2\varphi\end{bmatrix}=\begin{bmatrix}2xy\\x^2-y^2\end{bmatrix},\tag{32}$$

resulting in $3\times 8=24$ linear independent measurements. Having defined the measurement geometry, now the characteristic functions $\kappa_i(\vec{x})$ and the matrix $\mathbf{W}$ can be calculated from the eqs. (21,29), and $\mathbf{W}$ can be inverted.

As test field we choose

$$v_z(x,y)=\ln\frac{\left[(x-x_1)^2+(y-y_1)^2+b^2\right]}{\left[(x-x_0)^2+(y-y_0)^2+a^2\right]}+\ln\left(r_0{}^2\right)\quad\text{with}\tag{33}$$

$$\begin{bmatrix} x_0 \\ y_0 \end{bmatrix} = r_0 \begin{bmatrix} \cos \varphi_0 \\ \sin \varphi_0 \end{bmatrix}, \quad \begin{bmatrix} x_1 \\ y_1 \end{bmatrix} = \frac{1}{r_0} \begin{bmatrix} \cos \varphi_0 \\ \sin \varphi_0 \end{bmatrix}, \quad b = \frac{a}{r_0},$$

$$r_0 = 0.7, \quad \varphi_0 = 135°, \quad a = 0.5.$$

v_z vanishes at the pipe wall (physical constraint) and has an eccentric maximum. Its mesh and contour plot are depicted in Fig. 5 a. Fig. 3 shows the continuous potential distributions $U_0(\varphi)$, $U_1(\varphi)$, $U_2(\varphi)$, corresponding to the magnetic fields $\vec{B}_0$, $\vec{B}_1$, $\vec{B}_2$, and by the asterisks the voltages measured at the angles $\varphi = 0°, 45°, 90°, \ldots 315°$ are indicated.

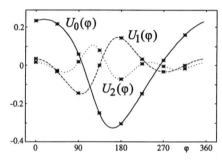

Fig. 3: Measured voltages.

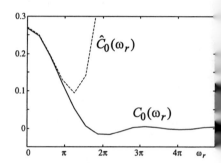

Fig. 4: Original (C_0) and approximated ($\hat{C}_0$) Fourier coefficients.

Now the reconstruction of $v_z(\vec{x})$ is straight forward: collecting the 24 voltages to a vector $\vec{u}$, multiplying $\vec{u}$ with $\mathbf{W}^{-1}$ (eq. (30)) and applying the adjoint operator $\mathcal{W}^*$ (eq. (31)). The result is shown in Fig. 5 b. Apart from some little deformations, the shape of the reconstructed velocity field, the location of the maximum, and the absolute values are met very well, related to the comparatively few number of 24 measurements. It should be emphasized, that the boundary values of the reconstructed field are zero, in agreement with the original field. This fact is due to the special weighting function $\varrho(\vec{x})$ of the inner product in $L_2^\varrho(\Omega)$, defined in eq. (20), which forces both the characteristic functions $\kappa_i(\vec{x})$ and the reconstructed velocity $\hat{v}_z(\vec{x}) = \mathcal{W}^*\vec{u} = \sum_{i=1}^m \kappa_i(\vec{x})\hat{u}_i$ to be zero at the boundary (eqs. (21,31)).

If, in contrast, the relations of the theoretical analysis in the second section are used for reconstruction, the results are not satisfying. According to Fig. 2, the first five Fourier coefficients of the voltages $U_0(\varphi)$, $U_1(\varphi)$ and $U_2(\varphi)$ (i. e. the moments $M_\nu\{c_k(r)\}$, $M_\nu\{d_k(r)\}$ of the velocity field, cf. eq. (11)) were calculated approximately by applying Fast Fourier Transform to the samples depicted in Fig. 3. With these moments, the Hankel transforms $C_k(\omega_r)$, $D_k(\omega_r)$ of eq. (18) were approximated by truncated power series; the dominant term $C_0(\omega_r)$ and its approximation $\hat{C}_0(\omega_r)$ are depicted in Fig. 4. Obviously, only low-frequency spectral components are estimated sufficiently correct. According to eq. (16) the $\hat{C}_k(\omega_r)$, $\hat{D}_k(\omega_r)$ are composed to the Fourier transform $V_z(\omega_x, \omega_y)$, and the reconstructed field $v_z(x,y)$

is obtained by inverse 2D-Fourier Transform. The result is depicted in Fig. 5 c; it is hardly similar to the original. To achieve better results with the analytical method, the higher-frequency spectral components must be determined, requiring a larger number of measurements, i.e. electrodes and magnetic fields.

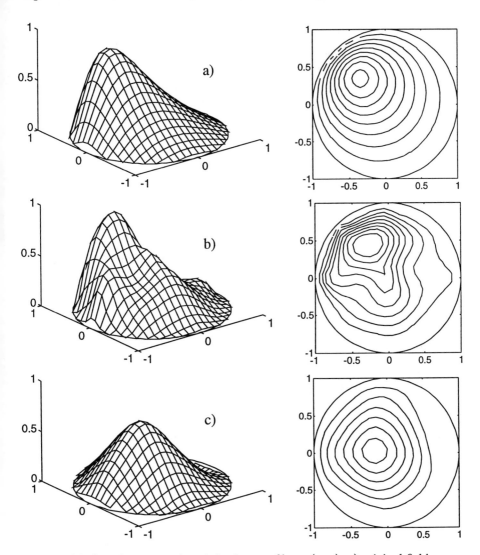

Fig. 5: Mesh and contour plot of the flow profiles $v_z(x, y)$: a) original field, b) Direct Algebraic Reconstruction, c) analytical reconstruction.

Table 2: Comparison of the reconstructions by performance indices.

	reconstruction with DAR	analytic reconstruction
E_1	3.201 %	11.1 %
E_2	5.682 %	19.7 %
$\max(\hat{v}_z)$	0.9267	0.6170

$\max(v_z) = 0.8409$

$$E_1 = \frac{\iint (\hat{v}_z - v_z)^2 \mathrm{d}^2 x}{\iint v_z{}^2 \mathrm{d}^2 x},$$

$$E_2 = \frac{\iint (\hat{v}_z - v_z)^2 \mathrm{d}^2 x}{\iint (v_z - \bar{v}_z)^2 \mathrm{d}^2 x},$$

$$\bar{v}_z = \frac{1}{\pi} \iint v_z \mathrm{d}^2 x.$$

In Table 2 the performance of the reconstructions is quantified by some performance indices confirming Fig. 5. All in all, DAR is clearly preferable because both measurement and reconstruction are appropriately formulated as mapping between the infinite-dimensional function space of the velocity field and the finite-dimensional vector space of measured data.

References

[1] B. Horner and F. Mesch, An Induction Flowmeter Insensitive to Asymmetric Flow Profiles, in Proceedings of ECAPT 95, ed. M.S. Beck et al. (UMIST. Manchester, 1995), pp. 321-330.

[2] F. Mesch, Sensing Principles and Reconstruction,. in this volume.

[3] T. Teshima, S. Honda and Y. Tomita, Electromagnetic Flowmeter with Multiple Poles and Electrodes, in Proceedings of IMTC 94 (Shizuoka, 1994).

[4] F. Natterer, Efficient Implementation of 'Optimal' Algorithms in Computerized Tomography, Math. Meth. in the Appl. Sci. 2 545-555 (1980).

[5] M.H. Buonocore, W.R. Brody and A. Macovski, A Natural Pixel Decomposition for Two-Dimensional Image reconstruction, IEEE Trans. Biomed. Eng. 28 69-78 (1981).

[6] A.C. Kak, M. Slaney, Principles of Computerized Tomographic Imaging. (IEEE Press, New York, 1987).

[7] J.A. Shercliff, The Theory of electromagnetic flow-measurement, (Cambridge, University Press, 1962).

[8] G. Schommartz, Induktive Strömungsmessung, (Verl. Technik, Berlin, 1974).

[9] P. M. Morse, H. Feshbach, Methods of Theoretical Physics, Part II, (Mc Graw-Hill, New York, 1953), p. 1188.

[10] A. Papoulis, Systems and Transforms with Applications in Optics, (Mc Graw-Hill, New York, 1968).

Part III

Applications

Chapter 15

Detecting Leaks in Hydrocarbon Storage Tanks Using Electrical Resistance Tomography

W. Daily and A. Ramirez
Lawrence Livermore National Laboratory
Livermore, California 94550 USA

D. LaBrecque
University of Arizona
Tucson, Arizona 85721 USA

A. Binley
Lancaster University
Lancaster, England LA1 4YQ U.K.

. Introduction

Large volumes of hydrocarbons are stored worldwide in surface and underground tanks. It is well documented [1] that all too often these tanks are found to leak, resulting in not only a loss of stored inventory but, more importantly, contamination to soil and groundwater. Two field experiments are reported herein to evaluate the utility of electrical resistance tomography (ERT) for detecting and locating leaks as well as delineating any resulting plumes emanating from steel storage tanks.

Current leak detection methods for single shell tanks require careful inventory monitoring, usually from liquid level sensors within the tank, or placement of chemical sensors in the soil under and around the tank. Liquid level sensors can signal a leak but are limited in sensitivity and, of course, give no information about the location or the leak or the distribution of the resulting plume. External sensors are expensive to retrofit and must be very densely spaced to assure reliable detection, especially in heterogeneous soils. The proposed method of subsurface tomography minimizes or eliminates these shortcomings.

The strategy of our approach as shown in Fig. 1 is to produce a tomograph of electrical resistivity under a storage tank and look for changes in the subsurface resistivity which could be attributed to spillage of the tank contents in the subsurface soil or groundwater. To test this strategy in a field demonstration, we would like to produce a tomograph of the soil under a tank and then, while observing changes of subsurface electrical properties, release the contaminant near the tank to simulate a leak. Unfortunately, this approach is not possible for many relevant liquids because laws protecting the environment prohibit intentional contamination even for research and development. Fortunately, the objectives of such research can be achieved by performing the work in two stages. For this reason the work described herein has been done in two parts. The first part of the work is to demonstrate that useful ERT images can be constructed in the soil beneath a large steel tank. The technical objective of this part is to produce images under a tank even when electrical currents are shunted away from the soil through the steel tank bottom. The purpose of the second experiment is to determine if a common liquid stored in tanks, gasoline, can be detected in the subsurface using ERT. The technical objective of this part is to determine if an electrically resistive liquid, floating on the groundwater, could be detected using electrical methods.

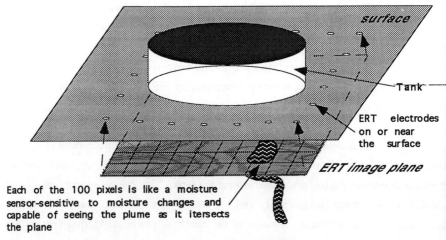

Figure 1. Schematic of leak detection concept using ERT.

2. Experimental Approach-tank leak imaging

The first phase is to demonstrate that useful ERT images can be constructed for the soil beneath a large steel tank. The field experiment was performed under a 15 m diameter steel tank mockup (the tank was not actually used for liquid storage). About 4000 liters of 0.08 molar sodium chloride solution were released along a portion of the tank's edge to simulate a leak from "bathtub ring" corrosion. The release rate averaged about 26 liters/hour. Fig. 2 shows the layout of the site where the experiments were performed.

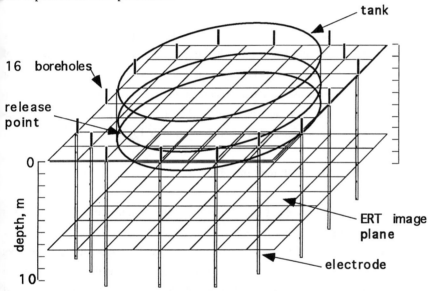

Figure 2. Schematic of experimental set up for leak detection. A 15 m diameter steel tank, the lower 2 meters of which is buried, contains a built-in spill point. Sixteen boreholes, with eight electrodes in each, surround the tank.

ERT images were made before, during and after the brine release in each of 8 horizontal planes beneath the tank. Plane 8 is a cross section at the ground surface 1.5 m above the bottom of the tank (so it contained the tank itself). Plane 7 is 1.5 m lower, a cross section level with the tank bottom. Plane 6 is 1.5 m below the tank bottom and so on to plane 1 which is 10.7 m below the ground surface. This arrangement provided a series of image planes at many levels which, when assembled together, gave an overall view of the plume formed beneath the tank during the release and which could be used to determine the effects of imaging current shunted through the tank bottom.

Data were collected in each plane before the release and then repeated for each plane at several times during and after the release. To simulate long term monitoring of a tank, we compared each data set taken during the release to a corresponding data set taken before the release. The comparison was done by inverting the quantity

$$\frac{R_a}{R_b} R_h$$

where R_a is the transfer resistance taken after the release, R_b is the transfer resistance taken before the release and R_h is the calculated transfer resistance for a model of uniform resistivity. The transfer resistance is simply the ratio of voltage to current for an individual 4 electrode measurement. This comparison is a simple perturbation from the uniform resistivity case as described in [2]. Other details of the data collection and inversion schemes are described by [2] and [3].

3. Experimental Results-tank leak imaging

Fig. 3 presents a series of two-dimensional tomographs collected from each electrode array at a given depth during the course of the release. The results show what areas of the soil changed in response to the brine spill. Each column of images shows the changes detected for a given time at various depths; the depth of images on each column increases from top (0 m depth) to bottom (10.7 m depth). Time and total released volume increase from left to right on the figure.

The images for July 26 at depths of 3 and 4.6 m show detectable electrical conductivity increases directly below the release point. The next day the anomaly is about a 20% resistivity change at 4.6 m depth. Note that the changes observed increase in magnitude as time and spilled volume increase. Also, note that the bottom of the changing region extends deeper as time increases. Electrical noise measurements were also made during the tests. These measurements where then used to calculate images which showed the magnitude of changes expected from measurement error only (these error images are not shown). The resistivity changes shown in Fig. 3 are substantially larger than those changes caused by measurement error. We conclude that the changes observed are caused by the released brine as it invades the soil.

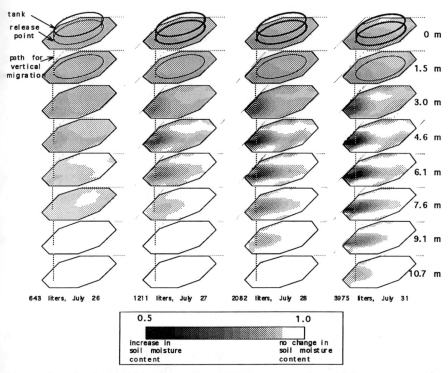

Figure 3. A series of two-dimensional ERT tomographs which show how the electrical conductivity of the soil increased during the side release experiment. White on the gray scale indicates which portions of the images remain unchanged. Shades of gray to the left on the scale indicate which portions of the image show electrical conductivity increases associated with the leak.

Although there are no corroborating data, the images are consistent with the behavior expected for infiltration of water released into a fairly homogeneous unsaturated soil. There is a clear decrease in resistivity of the volume directly below the release point from which the plume appears to drain downward by gravity and move laterally as it encounters soil heterogeneity. The approximate leak location can be found directly above the region of maximum change in the top few planes. The lateral and vertical extent of the plume as a function of time can also be estimated from the images.

4. Experimental Approach-gasoline plume imaging

The purpose of this phase was to determine if ERT could be used to image the location and extent of free product gasoline in the subsurface. This work was performed at the Oregon Graduate Institute of Science and Technology (OGI) in Beaverton, Oregon because the facilities there include a unique double-wall tank filled with soil into which a contaminant could be legally released at a scale sufficiently large to see real-world physical phenomena. The 10 m square and 5 m deep tank is instrumented for geophysical and hydrological studies. Sandy silt from river bottom sediments was randomly put into the tank; no effort was made to produce a structured fill (e.g., layers). Soil pore water was city water having a 0.004 S/m conductivity. A more complete description of the OGI facility can be found in [4].

Two boreholes in the tank were instrumented with electrodes and electrodes were installed on the surface between these holes. The reconstruction model assumes a resistivity distribution constant in the direction perpendicular to the plane defined by the electrodes although electrical potential is modeled three dimensionally to permit point electrodes. The soil-air interface is a boundary of zero normal current flow. After reconstruction, the tomographs are spatially smoothed to give the appearance of a continuous resistivity distribution. This, of course, doesn't improve resolution which can be no better than one mesh element. The mesh elements were approximately square and there were two elements between each electrode along the boreholes.

5. Experimental Results-gasoline plume imaging

A total of 408 liters of unleaded gasoline were released over an 81 hour period from August 28 through 31, 1992. This amounted to a rate of about 4 l/hr released from a single point on the surface midway between the boreholes. The phreatic surface was stable at a depth of 80 cm for several days before the release (the vadose zone had drained from saturated condition during these several days).

ERT data were taken before, several times during and again after the release. The data taken before the release were the intended baseline but were particularly noisy. Several artifacts appeared in the image especially at the electrode positions. Because of these errors, we found the 'before' image to be unsuitable as a baseline. The data taken after the release of only 40 liters of gasoline had much less noise and was used as the baseline for the release sequence.

Fig. 4 shows this August 28 baseline and subsequent pixel by pixel difference images. As early as August 30 we notice a definite resistive anomaly formed directly below the release point. It appears as a narrow anomaly from the surface downward and points to a larger anomaly which may be the main body of the plume at about the level of the original water saturated surface. The small anomaly pointed downward from the surface release point may be the barely resolved conduit from the surface to the point where the gasoline begins to spread in the capillary fringe. Such conduits are a common feature of large volume releases over short times and are called the descent cone by Farmer [5]. The larger anomaly below this descent cone represents a 15 - 20 percent increase in resistivity over the background values which is larger than anomalies caused by measurement error. We believe this resistive anomaly is caused by gasoline accumulation in the available vadose porosity in the vicinity of the water table.

The main anomaly on August 30, September 1 and September 2 is centered on the original water table. Because gasoline will float on or near the top of the capillary fringe, its influence should be confined predominately to the upper portion of the saturated zone. However, if the gasoline only displaces pore air in this water-wet system, one resistive fluid replaces another, and this should not significantly change the net resistivity. Any perturbation of electric current flow in the partially saturated soil must result from either a spatial redistribution of the water or a change in the electrical properties of the pendular water (that held by capillarity).

The mechanisms for either of these conditions are not clear. However one likely mechanism is a change in the capillary suction of water arising from the introduction of gasoline into the pore volume. This mechanism requires that the pendular water capillary suction change as a result of replacement of the air-water interface in the partially saturated pore with a hydrocarbon-water interface. Such a

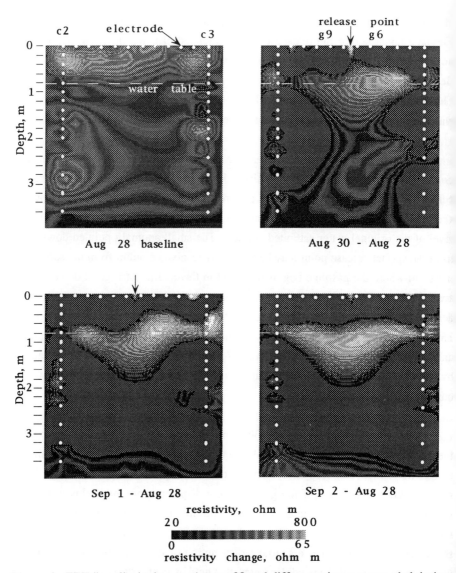

Figure 4. ERT 'baseline' taken on August 28 and difference images recorded during the gasoline release. The scale for the baseline image is shown at the top of the gray scale and that for the other images is at the bottom.

change in capillary suction would mean a redistribution of pore water with a subsequent change in electrical properties. Whatever the mechanism, we believe that

:he hydrocarbon caused a net dewatering of the regions where gasoline entered the
pore volume.

When the hydrocarbon reaches the capillary fringe, the relative permeability
:o the immiscible liquid declines and there is a tendency for lateral movement along
the top of the fringe. Domenico and Schwartz [6] state that when a large volume of
fluid reaches this point in a short time, the capillary fringe collapses (water drains
under gravity to the fully saturated zone) and depresses the water table. They point
out that the amount of depression depends on the quantity of product and its density
but the fluid spreads in a relatively thin layer in the upper part of the capillary fringe.
On the other hand, the ERT images imply a depressed water table and a relatively
thick product layer. The anomaly appears in both the unsaturated and previously
saturated portions of the soil. As described above, the mechanism for the electrical
anomaly is probably displacement of pore water in both cases. Where the soil is
water saturated, the gasoline with a specific gravity of 0.68, sinks to a level where
buoyancy supports the mass. This displacement of water produced a resistive
anomaly below the original water table.

On September 1 the anomaly appears larger in size and exhibits greater
electrical contrast. No additional gasoline was released between the September 1 and
September 2 images. The anomaly had not changed size on September 2 although
there is evidence that it became more uniform and lower in overall contrast. This may
be indicative of lateral spreading.

If the resistive anomaly represents the extent of a compact and continuous
mass (say a volume 0.5 m thick and 2 m square using the September 1 image) in a
soil of 20 percent available porosity (another assumption), we get a rough estimate of
the released volume of gasoline at the end of the release of 400 liters. Although this
is a simple analysis based on crude but plausible assumptions, the result compares
favorably with the 408 liters released.

6. Summary and Conclusions

The work described above has been done to determine the feasibility of using
ERT to detect and locate hydrocarbon leaks from large steel storage tanks. The

strategy is to produce an ERT image under a tank and look for changes in subsurface resistivity arising from leaks as a plume moves through the soil. A tomographic image beneath a tank can be constructed with data from a relatively few electrodes at or near the ground surface. However, each of the many pixels in that image acts as a separate leak sensor beneath the tank, greatly enhancing the ability to detect a leak.

Many of the tanks in question are of steel construction and contain hydrocarbon products. These facts define two principal issues requiring investigation. First, can useful ERT images be made near a highly conducting steel tank bottom or will all the current used for imaging be shunted through the steel making in impossible to image the soil under the tank? Second, will an electrically insulating hydrocarbon produce a change in subsurface resistivity in the vadose or saturated soil which can be imaged by ERT? These issues had to be addressed separately because of laws prohibiting the release of hydrocarbon into the ground.

In the first experiment, we demonstrate that useful images of changes in electrical resistivity can be produced near the bottom of a large steel tank. This is accomplished by inverting a normalized ratio of data taken before and after a release. Images delineate clearly a released tracer in reconstruction planes as close as a few meters from the tank bottom for anomalies greater than about 10% change in resistivity. However, we have not addressed complications such as cathodic protection systems used on tanks or natural subsurface seasonal variations. These effects will be studied in future work.

In the second experiment we have demonstrated that a common tank constituent, gasoline, will produce a change in subsurface resistivity which can be electrically imaged. Results suggest that an optimal case for electrical detection is when the hydrocarbon depresses the capillary fringe at the water table. For this case changes in resistivity of 15% to 20 % can be expected. However, we have little evidence for how the method would work in a completely unsaturated soil. Results from the controlled gasoline imaging would also likely be much different in a geologically complex environment.

These two experiments suggest that it may be possible to detect and locate leaks from tanks using ERT. While the work demonstrates feasibility of the

:echnique under the ideal, controlled circumstances available in these experiments, it does not prove the technique practical under more realistic conditions. Our work is continuing with the goal of studying the more realistic conditions caused by cathodic protection systems, infiltration of rain water, seasonal variation in the subsurface resistivity, contaminant type, variations in soil type and water table proximity.

7. References

[1]   R. M. Cohen and J. W. Mercer, <u>DNAPL Site Evaluation</u> (C. K. Smoley, 1993).

[2]   W. Daily, A. Ramirez, D. LaBrecque and J. Natio, Water Resources Research **28** 1429-1442 (1992).

[3]   D. J. LaBrecque, W. Daily, E. Owen, and A. Ramirez, "Noise and OCCAM's Inversion of Resistivity Tomography Data", Geophysics (in press, 1995).

[4]   R. L. Johnson, W. Bagby, M. Perrott, and C. Chen, in Proceedings of the 1992 Petroleum Hydrocarbons and Organic Chemicals in Ground Water: Prevention, Detection and Restoration (November 4-6, 1992, Houston, TX).

[5]   V. E. Farmer, "Behavior of Petroleum Contaminants in an Underground Environment", in Proc. Petroleum Assoc. for Conservation of the Canadian Environment (Ottawa, 1983).

[6]   P. A. Domenico and F. W. Schwartz, <u>Physical and Chemical Hydrogeology</u> (John Wiley, New York, 1990).

Acknowledgment
     This study is based on work performed under the auspices of the U. S. Department of Energy by the Lawrence Livermore National Laboratory under contract W-7405-ENG-48.

Chapter 16

Electrical Capacitance Tomography for Fluidized Bed Analysis

T. Dyakowski
Department of Chemical Engineering University of Manchester Institute of Science and Technology PO Box 88, Manchester M60 1QD

. Introduction

A knowledge of unsteady solid concentration is vital to characterize the dynamic behaviour of a fluidized bed. The flow pattern of the fluidized bed is determined by particle-particle, particle-gas interaction and bubble coalescence. These interactions, in a time domain, can therefore be characterized by both large and small scale fluctuations. The rapid fluctuations (over intervals of milliseconds or less) of voidage in the bed, normally negate the possibility of using radiation-based tomographic sensors, but such phenomena can be sensed using electrical methods. A typical mean size of a large air bubble is one tenth of the bed diameter and is thus in the range of the spatial resolution of recently developed, non-invasive, imaging methods, based on capacitance tomography, [1-4].

. Instrumentation

The multi-plane fluidized, bed tomographic system consists of three parts: the capacitive sensor, the sensor electronics and the computer or transputer networks, as shown in Fig. 1. The sensor developed by the Morgantown Energy Technology Centre was used to investigate the motion of the individual bubbles generated by an air pulse system and the aim of the UMIST system was to investigate the dynamic behaviour

of the fluidized bed, in the vicinity of the air distributor. The main characteristics of
the two systems are listed in Table 1.

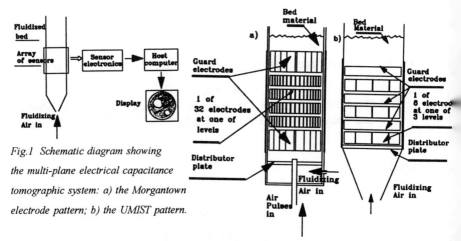

Fig.1 Schematic diagram showing
the multi-plane electrical capacitance
tomographic system: a) the Morgantown
electrode pattern; b) the UMIST pattern.

Table 1. Main characteristics of existing ECT systems

	System	
	Morgentown Energy Technology Centre	UMIST
Electronic circuit	AC − bridge	charge−discharge
Applied voltage [V]	500	15
Excitation frequency [MHz]	0.40	1.25
Measurement variable	Displacement current	Displacement current
Electrode configuration	4 sets 32 electrodes	3 sets 8 electrodes
Electrode area [m²]	3.3 • 10⁻⁴	18 • 10⁻⁴
Reconstruction algorithm	solving overdetermined system of equations	back projection
Number of pixels	193	1024
Rating rate [s⁻¹]	60	100

An electrical potential is applied to pairs of electrodes, which induces a
displacement current between electrodes. This current depends on the electrical
permittivity of the material between the electrodes. Assuming that the electrical
permittivity is proportional to the solid concentration, void fraction measurements can
be obtained. An instrument is calibrated using all-air and all-solids at a compacted
voidage, to establish the extremes of permittivity. The void fraction distribution is
characterized be the grey level of each individual pixel.

The capacitance between two electrodes is a function of both the permittivity of phases in the measurement volume and their distribution. The wave length of the generated electrical field is much larger than the diameter of the vessel. Therefore, any interrogated, fluidized bed process is governed by a solution of the electrostatic field equation. Neglecting the effect of electrical charges on particles, the electrical field between two electrodes is described by a Poisson equation:

$$\Delta \varphi(x,y) + \frac{1}{\varepsilon(x,y)} \nabla((\varphi(x,y)) \nabla(\varepsilon(x,y))) = 0 \qquad (1)$$

and the capacitance C between a pair of electrodes is described by the following formula:

$$C = -\frac{\iint_A \varepsilon(x,y) \nabla(\varphi(x,y)) dA}{\varphi_2 - \varphi_1} \qquad (2)$$

Deduction of the internal permittivity distribution, requires inversion from the set of boundary measurements. This amounts to image reconstruction from the boundary set of sensors. For an ECT system this reconstruction problem is strongly non-linear and ill posed. Therefore, a simplified method such as back projection is used to calculate, in a qualitative way, permittivity distribution. This method takes advantage of the fact that for most solids their dielectric permittivity is slightly larger than air permittivity, and thus is in the range 3-6. Therefore, as a first approach, it may be assumed that the distribution of an electrical field obtained for an all-air calibration is not affected by the solid's presence. This is a fundamental assumption lying behind the back projection method dealing with solving a Poisson equation. The grey level of the reconstructed image is expressed as:

$$G(x,y) = \frac{\sum\limits_{i=1}^{N-1} \sum\limits_{j=i+1}^{N} c_{i,j}(x,y) s_{i,j}(x,y)}{\sum\limits_{i=1}^{N-1} \sum\limits_{j=i+1}^{N} s_{i,j}(x,y)} \qquad (3)$$

where $c_{i,j}$ is the normalized capacitance measurements and $s_{i,j}$ the filed sensitivity distribution, of electrode pair i-j. $s_{i,j}$ is calculated from the following equation, by using a finite element method:

$$s_{i,j}(x,y) = -\frac{1}{V_i V_j} \int\limits_{p(x,y)} \vec{E}_i(x,y) \cdot \vec{E}_j(x,y) dx dy \qquad (4)$$

where E_i (x,y) is the electrical field distribution when electrode i is the source electrode (applied with a positive potential V_i) while other electrodes E_j (x,y) are at earth potential V_j; p(x,y) is the area of a pixel at (x,y).

3. Results and discussion

Heat and mass transfer processes within a fluidized bed mainly depend on the bubble coalescence mechanism. By using an ECT system, the images of the voidage distribution in a pipe cross section, as well along the height of the bed, can be obtained. These images allow for a description of the bubble coalescence mechanism and may also be used to measure a bubble rise velocity. Especially, can useful information be extracted from the images. This would be concerned with an order of magnitude of temporal and spatial scales, characterizing both convection and diffusion processes within the fluidized bed.

3.1 Flow regimes

The instantaneous voidage distribution for three flow regimes is shown in Fig. 2. A change in the flow pattern occurs in a transition from a slugging to a turbulent flow, Fig.2c. In the transition regime the centre of the pipe cross-section is occupied by the air stream. For this flow regime the wall attached bubbles were not observed, as they were for the two previous flow regimes. The corresponding concentration maps given below each isometric plot show white regions indicating the area occupied by air.

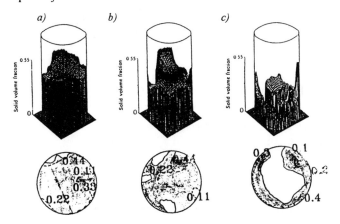

Fig.2 Isometric solid volume fraction distribution and corresponding concentration maps for three different flow regimes: a) bubbling fluidization; b) slugging regime, and c) transition from a slugging to a turbulent regime.

3.2 Bubble coalescence

The process of bubble coalescence, for a slugging flow regime, is presented in Fig.3. For bubbling fluidization predominantly, bubbles were visible, attached to the walls and this is congruent with the results presented in [1]. However, it should be noted also that the spatial resolution of a capacitance system is lowest near the pipe centre, therefore, small bubbles appearing in the central pipe region may not be sensed. The white area, marked by I, corresponds to the bubble leaving the control volume. As shown, area II is almost constant. This is a consequence of a small time interval $\Delta t = 4.76$ ms between subsequent images. A large change in the area occupied by bubble II is caused by bubble II coalescing with bubble III entering the control volume.

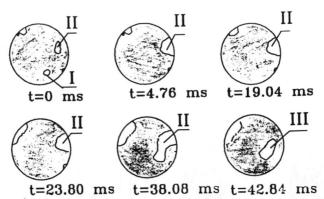

II   **II**   **II**

t=0 ms   t=4.76 ms   t=19.04 ms

II   **II**   **III**

t=23.80 ms   t=38.08 ms   t=42.84 ms

Fig.3 Time sequence of voidage distribution for a slugging flow regime. I-denotes a bubble leaving the control volume; II- denotes a bubble entering the control volume; III- denotes an area occupied by two bubbles after coalescing.

Below, two dimensional Eulerian slices or voidage contour plots are constructed, taking the horizontal co-ordinate along one of the tube diameters, on a light to dark scale. At any point in time, frames that are higher up, occurred earlier. Fig.4 illustrates an Eulerian slice of a void. The light area represents regions of higher voidage. Analyzing two-dimensional Eulerian slices, various types of bubble coalescence processes can be distinguished and appear as being explosive , draining or condensing, as shown in Fig.4.

a)   *Level 1*   *Level 2*   *Level 3*   *Level 4*

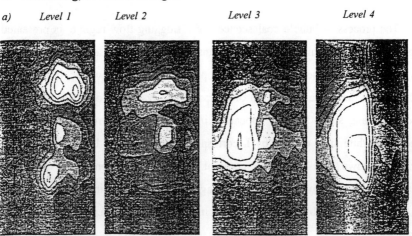

[Figure caption - over]

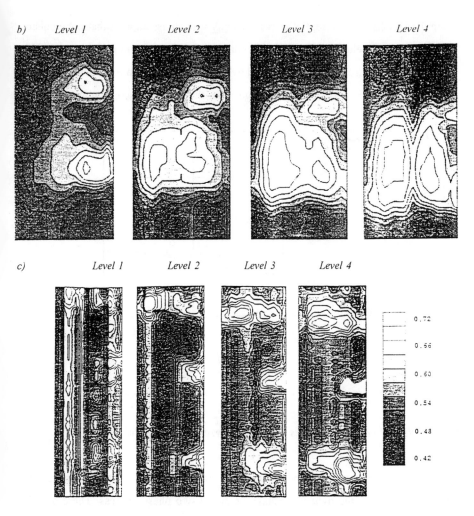

Fig.4 Eulerian slices illustrating various bubble coalescence mechanisms : a) explosive coalescence; b) draining, and c) condensing (after [1]).

3.3 Bubble rise velocity

A bubble rise velocity can be calculated by analyzing the images obtained from a multi-plane ECT system. The effect of the excess air velocity (superficial air velocity minus minimum fluidization air velocity) to reduce the data scatter as was proposed by Davidson and Harrison [6] was validated by [1]. It was shown that the main drawbacks of a concept of excess velocity was an assumption that the emulsion phase interstitial velocity is constant at minimum fluidization and neglects the bubble coalescence processes. This is confirmed by the results shown in Fig.5 which indicate that the bubble velocity is 2-3 times larger than the non-coalescing bubbles.

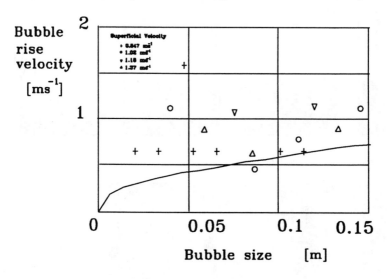

Fig.5 A bubble rise velocity as a function of the bubble size (after [1]).

3.4 Statistical coherence zones and cross-correlation velocity

The correlation functions measured in either space, or in time and space, are useful for defining the dynamic behaviour of the two phase process. Therefore, the spatial correlation of data across the image plane of the capacitance sensor (Fig.1b) is considered. Fig.6a shows the distribution of the normalized cross-correlation function between data at the centre of the bed and the image data at all pixels, away from the centre. The high values of this function (>0.7) are close to the centre of the bed and have a scale of rather less than half of the bed diameter. Fig.6b shows the distribution of the same function for data at the pipe wall and all pixels away from the pipe wall. High values of this function (>0.7) are close to the pipe bed wall. Therefore, the wall coherence zone is an annulus of approximately one fifth of the bed diameter.

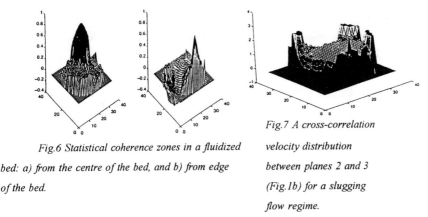

Fig.6 Statistical coherence zones in a fluidized
bed: a) from the centre of the bed, and b) from edge
of the bed.

Fig.7 A cross-correlation
velocity distribution
between planes 2 and 3
(Fig.1b) for a slugging
flow regime.

As was discussed above, a free rise velocity of a single bubble does not fully represent the movement of excess air. The velocity of excess air can be characterized by a cross-correlation velocity which measures how the voidage distribution, statistical in nature, is 'moved' along the bed height. This velocity calculated for each pixel is shown in Fig.7

3.5 Deterministic chaos approach

There is experimental evidence [2], [5], that a fluidized bed is a chaotic system with stochastic dynamics which can be characterized by two time scales: large scale fluctuations occur due to the formation of bubbles during fluidization, caused by the circulating motion of the particles, small fluctuations are induced by interphase interaction between individual particles or collections of particles. To explain the deterministic behaviour of the fluidized bed, a theoretical model based on a single chain of bubbles moving along the bed axis, was proposed by [2]. In this model the distances between bubbles were described by a set of nonlinear ordinary differential equations. To define the overall state of the system, the co-ordinates of the bubbles have to be calculated. The number of bubbles, and thus the number of equations in the chain model, changes with time. The main drawback of this model is that it neglects bubble movements and interaction in a radial direction. Nevertheless, it can be used as a first step for simulating the dynamic behaviour of a fluidized bed. The results of a numerical simulation and experimental data are shown in Fig.8.

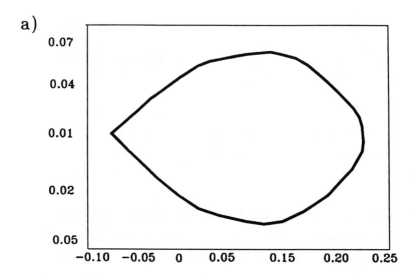

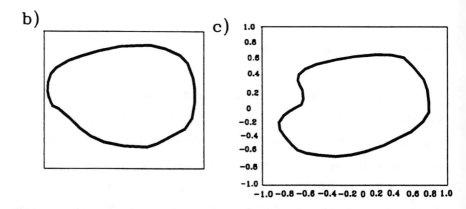

Fig.8 The shape of strange attractors illustrating the dynamic behaviour of a fluidized bed: a) calculated in [2]; b) measured on a basis of the pressure fluctuations [5]; c) measured on a basis of the voidage distribution.

For multiple periodic motions, the power spectrum consists only of discrete lines of corresponding frequencies, whereas chaotic motion (which is completely aperiodic) is indicated by a broad noise $P(\omega)$ that is most intense at low frequencies. A spectrum analysis is presented in Fig.9.

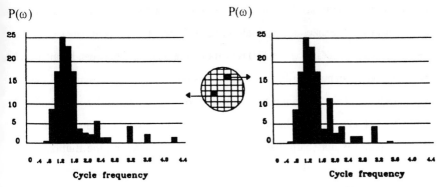

Fig.9 Power spectrum of two signals measured at two different pixel location.

The Kolomogorov entropy K which measures 'how chaotic a dynamic system is,' can be defined by Shannon's formula in such a way that K becomes proportional to the rate at which information about the state of the dynamic system is lost in the course of time. K becomes zero for regular motion, it is infinite in random systems, but is a constant larger than zero if the systems display deterministic chaos. According to [2],[5] the value of the K entropy is in the range 2-15.

4. Conclusion

The existing ECT systems for imaging the fluidized bed behaviour differ significantly in electronic circuits, number of electrodes as well as reconstruction algorithm. 500 volts are needed to excitate a Morgantown system and 15 volts are needed for the UMIST system. A Morgantown system has 32 electrodes sitting inside the pipe and the UMIST system has only 8 which are fixed at the outer surface. For nearly the same pipe diameter, there are 193 pixels in a Morgantown system and 1024 pixels in the UMSIT system. Both systems have an excellent temporal resolution below 0.015 s. The spatial resolution of the Morgantown system is below 7% of the pipe diameter and for the UMIST system it is around 10%.

It is demonstrated that this tomographic technique is capable of providing a substantial amount of data on the temporal and spatial variations in bed voidage.

These allow quantification of the bubble-particle interaction dynamics and enable visualization of bubble size, shape, coalescence etc. The results concerned with the bubble coalescence processes (Figs 2-4) reveal that the boundary between bubbles and an emulsion phase can be described as a 'fuzzy boundary' with the presence of a large voidage gradient. This is congruent with the results obtained by using X-ray photography [7]. On the other hand, the fact that the boundary between bubbles and an emulsion phase is not sharp, has a strong impact on modelling the fluidized bed behaviour. A main drawback of existing theoretical models is an assumption that a boundary surface in the fluidized bed is as uniquely defined as in a gas-liquid flow.

The results show that an ECT system can be used to construct and validate the fluidized bed model based on a deterministic chaos theory. The shapes of the calculated strange attractors have been compared with independently experimentally obtained results data from the Morgantown Centre, Delft University and UMIST; agreement with the numerical prediction is good. In future, a two dimensional model taking into account the bubble movement in the radial direction can be developed. Such a model should allow for the description of both convection and diffusion processes within a fluidized bed.

5. References

[1]   J.S. Halow and P.Nicoletti Powder Technology **69** 255-277 (1992)

[2]   C.S. Daw and J.S. Halow A.I.Ch.E. Symp. 289 **88** 61-69 (1992)

[3]   J.S. Halow, G.E. Fasching and P. Nicoletti A.I.Ch.E. Symp. 276 **86** (1990)

[4]   S.J. Wang, T. Dyakowski, C.G. Xie, R.A. Williams and M.S. Beck The Chemical Engineering Journal **56** 95-100 (1995)

[5]   C.M. van den Bleek and J.C. Schouten The Chemical Engineering Journal **53** 75-87 (1993)

[6]   J.F. Davidson and D.Harrison, Fluidized Particles, (Cambridge University Press, New York, 1963)

[7]   J.G. Yates, D.J. Cheesman and Y.A. Sergeev Chemical Eng. Sci. **49** 12 1885-1895 (1994)

Chapter 17

Gamma Ray Imaging of Industrial Fluidized Beds

J. R. Bernard[1], L. Desbat[2], and P. Turlier[1]

[1] Unite Mixte ELF-CNRS Catalytic Engineering of Refining Reactors
Centre de Recherche ELF, B.P. 22 Solaize 69360 FRANCE

[2] Faculté de Médecine, Université J. Fourier
La Tronche 38706 FRANCE

1. Applications of Fluidized Beds

A fluidized bed is formed by flowing a fluid (often a gas) through a bed of solid particles. When the pressure drop due to the gas-solid friction is equal or larger than the weight divided by the bed area, the solid is fluidized and behaves like a liquid: it can flow, its density is proportional to differential pressure, gas may bubble in it and particles mix well. These interesting properties are used in a large number of processes where bulk solid handling would be too costly.

For instance, fluidized beds were developed for coal combustion, thus allowing the continual withdraw of ashes and taking advantage of the good heat transfer capabilities of the bed. In the oil industry, fluidized catalytic cracking plants (FCC, Fig. 1) convert heavy feedstocks to provide 50% of the gasoline market. In this process, the catalyst is continuously circulated through pipes and valves between a reactor where it deactivates and a regenerator where it is regenerated. There are many other fluidized bed processes, mainly in the chemical industry where fluidization is used to control exothermic reactions like catalytic selective oxidation. The development and even the daily operation of these plants is sometimes not simple and the knowledge of their internal operation is useful. The purpose of this chapter is to show how gamma ray tomography is designed and used within the ELF AQUITAINE group to inspect its FCC plants.

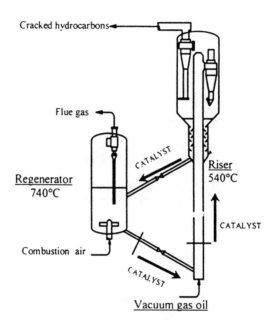

Fig. 1 Typical Fluid Catalytic Cracking Plant

2. History of Fluidized Beds Tomography

Like Rowe with his X ray device designed to study bubbles [1], chemical engineers took advantage of the progress in medical imaging diagnostic to obtain local information on small fluidized beds [2]. The main limitation of X rays use is their high absorption which limits the bed size. Capacitance tomography is probably more adapted to cold beds when they can have non conductive walls. Pictures can be obtained with a good resolution from a quite simple and safe device and bed instabilities can be detected. By contrast, industrial beds walls are always metallic and sometimes refractory lined. The only possibility to get information from non-invasive techniques is the use of high energy ionizing radiation, i.e., gamma rays. The first gamma tomography experiment by Bartholomew and Casagrande [3] described in 1957 refers to a 0.51m I.D. FCC riser with a 60Co source and a Geiger Mueller detector. The 18 paths layout was fan-beam shaped. The Radon transform was solved by assuming a 4th order polynomial density function and determining its coefficients by the least squares method. As this required "considerable machine calculation time", a graphical method was also used. One month later, Hunt et al. [4] described a set up with 22 parallel paths with the same solving procedures. Two later publications [5,6] showed the use of gamma rays tomography to map fluidized catalyst density but no more information was given about the methods.

3. Physics of Gamma Ray Absorption

3.1 *Gamma source requirements*

Gamma photons can be completely absorbed by electrons (photoelectric effect) or they can diffuse by partial absorption (Compton effect). In this latter case, there is a spectrum of diffused photon energy which depends on the source energy, on the absorbing material and on the direction. These effects can be described by the Beer Lambert law

$$\frac{I}{I_0} = \exp\left(-\Sigma\rho\mu x\right)$$

where the mass absorption coefficient μ is representative of the photoelectric effect. This very short description indicates that directly applying this law without care may lead to large mistakes especially if the Compton effect is important.

Figure 2 shows photoelectric m as a function of photon energy. Below 100 keV, it is very sensitive to the elemental composition of the bed and it is more desirable to work with a more energetic source, say above 200 keV. Nevertheless, low energy sources can be used with gas fluidized beds when the solid composition does not vary, since gas density is often negligible. Source energy must also be adapted to the bed size and density to obtain good accuracy. For example, if the average bed density is 300 kg/m^3, the absorption half-length is 8 cm at 60 keV and 23 cm at 600 keV. Thus the smaller the bed, the less energetic the source required to maintain accuracy. Table 1 shows the properties of some typical radioisotopes.

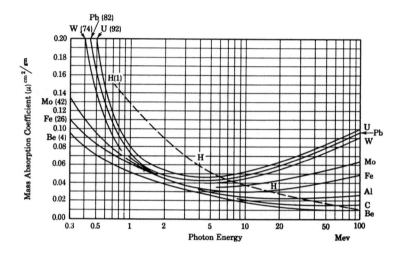

Fig. 2 Mass Absorption Coefficient of Gamma Rays

Radioisotope	Energy (keV)	Halflife (years)
Americium 241	60	432
Selenium 75	97 - 401	0.33
Barium 133	81, 276, 303, 356	10.5
Iridium 192	316 - 1061	0.20
Caesium 137	662	30
Gadolinium 153	69, 97, 103	0.66
Cobalt 60	1173, 1332	5.27

Table 1: Radioisotopes

In practice, we are using Americium for small dilute beds (I.D. 0.2 m) with perspex walls and Cs or Co for industrial beds (I.D ~1m) with steel walls. Radiographers are currently evaluating welds with Ir but its wide energy spectrum does not favour its use for quantitative measurements.

Once energy is defined, activity remains to be determined. Required accuracy becomes the key parameter to determine source activity. Radioactivity is a random process which obeys Poisson's law, and in the case of strong absorption, background noise must also be taken in consideration. If counting time is to be minimized, the highest possible activity must be chosen.

A final consideration is radioactivity protection. Strict rules are applied to protect personnel. There are maximum admissible radioactivity doses which limit source energy-activity and determine the characteristics of the lead container. For example non-specialized people may work with a 0.5 Ci Caesium source, but the container weighs 20 kg, which may be an upper limit for a versatile device. This limit determines the maximum vessel size that can be reasonably processed, i.e. between 1 and 2 m, depending on the density of the materials and the allowed sampling time.

3.2 *Gamma ray detection*

Scintillation counters are preferred to Geiger Mueller counters because of their better sensitivity, accuracy and stability. The size of the doped sodium iodide crystal must be chosen as a function of the scanning program to avoid any beam overlapping, otherwise detector saturation may occur.

Compton effects must be minimized as much as possible to avoid interferences from materials outside the direct beam. This is done by setting the discriminator on the data acquisition unit to a minimum energy level of detection to eliminate low energy scattered radiation. This is not always sufficient and detector collimation is also required at higher energies. It is in fact impossible to detect only unscattered rays unless collimation becomes so severe that problems of accuracy and positioning predominate. A good compromise must be found, but the consequence of scattering is that the Beer Lambert law cannot be used to model wall absorption and another scan must be done on the empty bed.

4. Scanning Program and Mathematics

The scanning program is imposed by the time available to do it. As the result is time averaged, it is essential to have an operation as steady as possible. A reasonable duration in our industry is 2-3 hours. A minimum sampling time of 20 s is required to obtain a time averaged density on the considered path because of hydrodynamic fluctuations. Depending on counting rate, each sampling may last up to several minutes. so that the number of measurements is limited to a few hundred. The problem is to optimize the placement of these measurements in order to get a best estimate of the solution (the image).

Tomographic concepts described in the literature [7] were adapted by Desbat [8,9]. Because of the small number of data, algebraic reconstruction is preferred. Interlaced sampling schemes are preferred to the usual standard schemes since they are theoretically twice as efficient. In this case, the optimum number of rotations is $p/2$ times the number of translations. However the advantage is partly lost because this configuration demands a better accuracy (signal to noise, positioning) which cannot always be satisfied. Currently an interlaced scheme of 18 rotations and 11 translations is used to map our industrial fluidized beds.

5. Practical Problems

The scanning apparatus must be as versatile and compact as possible, and it must ensure the best positioning reproducibility for several scans. In effect, a blank measurement on the empty pipe is necessary to account for the walls. This measurement must be done when the plant is shut down, sometimes several months or years later. Positioning reproducibility is a key point when working on a FCC riser. Usually most of the catalyst is accumulated near the walls and its density is low compared to the wall density (40 to 150 kg/m^3 for the catalyst versus 8000 kg/m^3 for steel). The closer the measurements are to the inside wall, the more important the wall contribution to the absorption becomes and the more delicate the operation is in terms of positioning and counting accuracy. The problem is often complicated by the presence of an internal concrete lining for thermal insulation and anti-erosion purposes.

6. Experimental Results

We applied the techniques described above to the study of FCC plants. The method is restricted to risers and standpipes since beds like those found in regenerators or strippers are too large for gamma ray inspection.

6.1 *Riser inspection*

Risers are the reactors where fast cracking reactions take place on contacting hydrocarbons and fluidized catalyst powder. The local performance of the catalyst in terms of reaction rate is proportional to the catalyst density and inversely proportional to the gas velocity. These two factors are connected by the relation:

catalyst density = (catalyst mass flux)/(gas velocity - gas_solid slip velocity)

since catalyst is entrained by gas. It can be concluded that if hydrocarbons and catalyst are not evenly distributed on the riser cross section, some diametrical gradients of conversion and yields may develop so that reactor performance is affected. Tomography and other techniques were used to investigate these phenomena on an industrial scale. Figure 3 shows a density map obtained from a 3x9 tomography of a 0.85m I.D. riser with a solid mass flux of 1090 kg/m^2/s and a gas velocity estimated at 25 m/s. Figure 4 shows another 18x11 tomography of a 0.79 I.D. riser with a mass flux of 590 kg/m^2/s and a gas velocity estimated to be 8 m/s. This information combined with momentum profiles obtained on a riser diameter allow us to obtain local catalyst flux and velocity.

6.2 *Standpipe inspection*

The standpipe is used to transfer fluidized catalyst by gravity from one vessel to another which can be at lower pressure. We present in Fig. 5 a 5x11 tomography of a 0.72 m I.D. 45° sloped standpipe with a 970 kg/m^2/s catalyst flux. Density is expressed relative to the solid bulk density. It appears in this case that catalyst is not fluidized close to the lower generatrix as it remains fluidized in the remaining part of the cross section, with probably some bubbles flowing in the upper part. The problems of

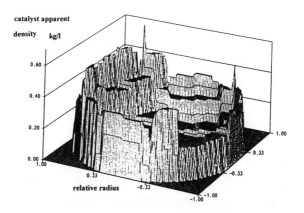

Fig. 3 Riser Tomography (3 rotations, 11 translations)

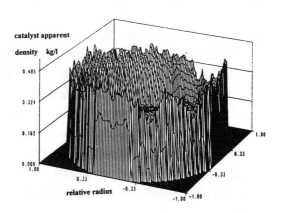

Fig. 4 Riser Tomography (18 rotations, 11 translations)

positioning accuracy and wall influence are not so severe in this case because catalyst concentration is much higher than in risers.

7.   Conclusions

Gamma ray tomography is currently the only tool which enables local density measurements in industrial fluidized beds. There are however limitations: size of the vessel, time averaged data, necessity to do a blank experiment. Moreover it is difficult to design a universal tomography system because needs and constraints differ from one site to an other. In some cases, a good wall model would represent a big step forward in the rapid acquisition of density maps.

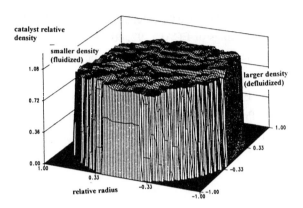

Fig. 5 Standpipe Tomography (5 rotations, 11 translations)
Density is relative to the apparent bulk density of the catalyst.

References

[1]   P. N. Rowe and C. Yacono, Trans. Inst. Chem. Engineers **53** 59-60 (1975).

[2]   W. F. Banholzer, C. L. Spiro, P. G. Kosty, and D.H. Maylotte, Ind. Eng. Chem. Res. **26** 763-767 (1987).

[3]   R. N. Bartholomew and R. M. Casagrande, Ind.Eng.Chem. **49** 428-431 (1957).

[4]   R. H. Hunt, W. R. Biles, and C. O. Reed, Petroleum Refiner **36** 179-182 (1957).

[5]   A. L. Saxton and A. C. Worley, The Oil and Gas Journal, May 18, 1970 82-98

[6]   H.G. Myers, Chemtech, August 1981, 489-492.

[7]   F. Natterer, The Mathematics of Computerized Tomography (Wiley, Chichester, 1986)

[8]   L. Desbats and P. Turlier, in Tomographic Techniques for Process Design and Operation, Proceedings of ECAPT '92, ed. M. S. Beck et al. (Computational Mechanics Publications, Southampton, 1993) pp. 285-294.

[9]   L. Desbats and P. Turlier, in Process Tomography - A Strategy for Industrial Exploitation, Proceedings of ECAPT '93, ed. M. S. Beck et al. (UMIST, Manchester, 1994) pp. 342-345.

Chapter 18

Quantitative X-Ray Computed Tomography and Its Application in the Process Engineering of Particulate Systems

J. D. Miller and C. L. Lin
Department of Metallurgical Engineering
University of Utah
Salt Lake City, Utah 84112, U.S.A.

Introduction

X-ray computed tomography (CT) had its origin in the medical sciences [1] and is now being used for non-medical and industrial applications [2]. Of course CT techniques generally have the unique advantage of providing detailed images of the internal structures of opaque materials in a non-destructive manner. Most of the industrial applications of CT are qualitative in nature, probably a carry-over from its use in the medical field. Nevertheless, it is important to note that CT images contain enough information to allow for quantitative analysis in the process engineering of particulate systems.

After a short description of the theoretical aspects of X-ray CT and the algorithm necessary for image reconstruction two applications of quantitative CT analysis are discussed. The first application is the use of CT for the examination of multiphase flow in air-sparged hydrocyclone flotation and the second application is the use of X-ray CT for coal washability analysis.

2. X-Ray Computed Tomography

2.1. *Basic Principles*

The basic principles of CT are well documented [1,3,4] and only a short over view is presented herein. The relationship between the initial intensity of an X-ray beam as it leaves the source and the final intensity of the same beam after it has passe through a section of the target material can be described by the following equation.

$$I_f = I_i e^{-\int_{Ray} \mu(x,y)\,ds}$$

(1

where:

I_i = initial intensity of the X-ray beam
I_f = final intensity of the X-ray beam
μ = linear attenuation coefficient.

Figure 1 illustrates the above mentioned equation [5].

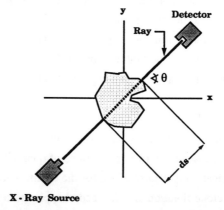

Fig. 1. A diagram showing an X-ray beam as it emanates from the source, passes
through the sample, and finally is collected at the detector [5].

An important assumption that was made implicitly in eq. (1) is that the X-ray beam intensity is monochromatic in nature. This is not strictly true. After rearrangement of eq. (1) in the following manner,

$$\log\left[\frac{I_i}{I_f}\right] = \int_{Ray} \mu(x, y)\, ds \qquad (2)$$

he left-hand side of eq. (2) represents the measured quantity. This value can be obtained from the CT machine. The right-hand side of eq. (2) is the ray integral of the -ray beam that passed through the sample. If *Ray* is defined as follows:

$$Ray = x\cos\theta - y\sin\theta \qquad (3)$$

hen the line integral can be written in the following manner.

$$P_\theta(Ray) = \int_{Ray} f(x, y)\, ds \qquad (4)$$

where:
  $P_\theta(Ray)$ is the projection of the X-ray beam that passed through the sample.

Notice that the right-hand side of eq. (4) is essentially the same as the right-hand side of eq. (2). The unknown function $f(x,y)$ simply takes the place of the linear attenuation function $\mu(x,y)$. By using the definition of the Dirac delta function, eq. (4) can be reformulated as:

$$P_\theta(Ray) = \int_{-\infty}^{\infty}\int_{-\infty}^{\infty} f(x, y)\, \delta(x\cos\theta - y\sin\theta - Ray)\, dx\, dy$$
$$(5)$$

Eq. (5) is known as the Radon transform of the function $f(x,y)$ which is the foundation of CT technology. The Radon transform provides the mathematical basis for the relationship between the projected data and the image reconstruction. If we pass a series of line integrals through the unknown function $f(x,y)$ at a fixed angle θ, we obtain what is called a projection $P(\theta)$ as shown in Figure 2 [5].

$P(\theta)$ can be obtained by using an assembly of sources and detectors and translating them at predefined intervals until they cover the entirety of the sample being

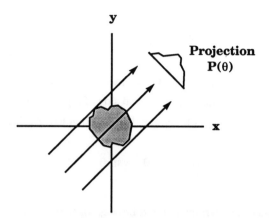

Fig. 2. An illustration showing several rays traversing through the sample at a fixed
angle. The data from the series of rays are called a projection $P(\theta)$ [5].

scanned. In order to use the projection $P(\theta)$ data to reconstruct an X-ray CT image, we
need to solve the Radon transform equation, i.e. eq. (5). Detailed mathematical algo
rithms for image reconstruction from the projection data based on the geometry of the
CT equipment can be found in standard texts [1,3,4].

In practice, one of the procedures for obtaining the reconstructed image from
CT projection data is shown in Figure 3 [5]. The first step is to collect the projection
data from the CT machine. The next step is to perform a convolution between the projection data and a suitable filter. The filtered projection is then back-projected to obtain
the reconstructed image. Additional image processing techniques such as thresholding
can be applied to obtain more pleasing images.

2.2. Advanced Reconstruction Algorithm

In order to obtain more accurate reconstruction of tomographic images, a new
algorithm is being developed [6]. This algorithm draws from the strength of the filtered back-projection method but is iterative in nature. This approach allows for the
inclusion of *a priori* information into the solution. A block diagram of the unit operations involved in the algorithm is shown in Figure 4. The basic steps in the new algorithm are as follows:

Steps in the Construction of a CT Image

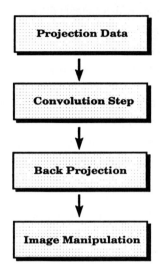

Fig. 3. A block diagram showing the steps necessary in the construction of an image obtained from a CT scanner [5].

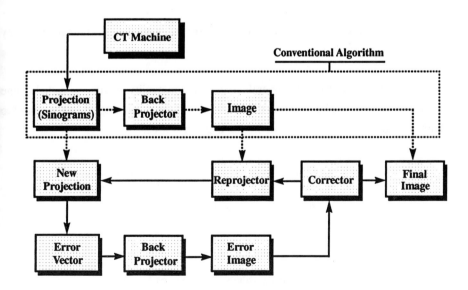

Fig. 4. A block diagram showing the various operations of the advanced algorithm. The operations enclosed in the dotted rectangle represent operations that are present in the conventional CT reconstruction algorithm [6].

1.   Obtain the projection data (sinograms) from the CT machine.
2.   Convolve the projections with a suitable filter.
3.   Perform the back-projection.
4.   Normalize the resulting image.
5.   Use a synthetic projector to create a new set of projection data from the reconstruction image.
6.   Compare the new set of projection data with the original data from step 1.
7.   Generate a set of error vectors.
8.   Back-project the generated error vectors to form an error image.
9.   Combine the error image with the original image to create a corrected image. If satisfied terminate the iteration, otherwise go back to step 5.

The unit operations enclosed in the dashed-lined block represent the steps normally present in a conventional CT reconstruction. All other unit operations shown represent enhancements that are introduced by the new algorithm.

The effectiveness of the new algorithm was tested by performing a numerical simulation. The simulation pattern consisted of three concentric squares with densities of 4.0 g/cc, 2.0 g/cc and 8.0 g/cc for outermost, middle and innermost squares, respectively [6]. The test pattern was chosen so that streaks emanating from the high-density square could be easily seen.

In order to quantify the overall reconstruction quality, a criterion called image error was defined. This represents the "distance" of the reconstructed image from the known original test pattern. The definition is given below.

$$Image \ \ Error \ = \ \sqrt{\frac{(original \ \ image - reconstructed \ \ image)^2}{original \ \ image^2}} \qquad (6)$$

where.

original image = the density values of the test pattern, and
reconstructed image = the density values of the reconstructed image.

Table 1 presents the image errors calculated from a conventional filtered backrojection algorithm and from the new algorithm. The number of iterations used was ree. The results show that the new algorithm was able to reduce the reconstruction rror by a factor of 2.

Table 1.Comparison of image errors obtained from the conventional filtered back-projection method and from the new algorithm after 3 iterations

	Conventional	New Algorithm
Image Error	0.0791	0.0328

3. Multiphase Flow Analysis - Air Sparged Hydrocyclone (ASH) Flotation

The air-sparged hydrocyclone (ASH) is distinguished by its high-specific capacity for fine particle flotation in a centrifugal field. To elaborate, it is now evident that the ASH has a specific capacity of at least 100 times that of conventional flotation equipment. The concept of ASH technology for fine particle flotation is based on the proposition that the energy for the inertial collision between a fine particle and an air bubble will be increased sufficiently in a strong centrifugal force field to achieve film rupture, bubble attachment and flotation. In ASH flotation the centrifugal force field is generated by conversion of pressure head into the rotational motion of swirl flow.

A schematic diagram of the air-sparged hydrocyclone is shown in Figure 5. The main features of the ASH are a porous tube through which air is sparged and a tangential flow of the particle suspension orthogonal to the air flow. The suspension passes downward through the ASH in swirl flow and a counter-current flow of the froth phase moves upward and towards the center of the device. Hydrophilic particles are thrown against the porous tube wall by the centrifugal field and are discharged through the annular underflow opening. Hydrophobic particles encounter the air bubbles which are sparged radially through the porous tube. Particle/bubble attachment occurs, and the hydrophobic particles are transported into the froth phase which exits axially at the top of the cyclone through a vortex finder [7-9].

Understanding of the flow behavior has been limited due to experimental difficulties associated with the presence of the opaque, inner porous tube of the ASH. Conventional measurement techniques such as high-speed photography and laser Doppler anemometry are difficult to use. In order to gain a better understanding of how

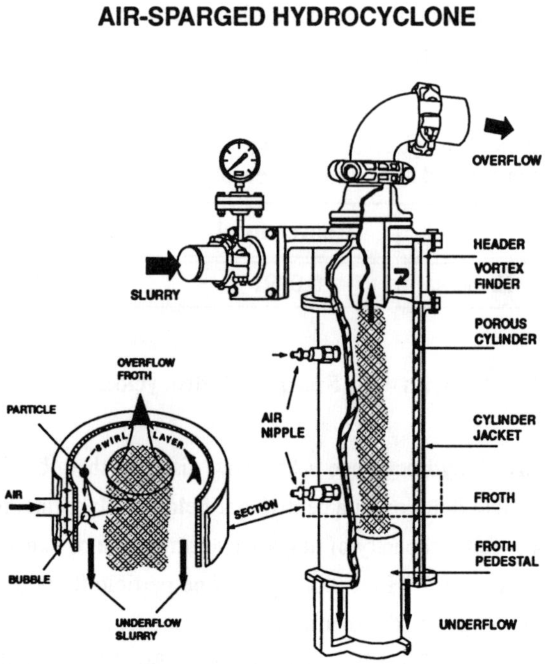

AIR-SPARGED HYDROCYCLONE

Fig. 5. A perspective drawing of the air-sparged hydrocyclone (ASH).

different particles are distributed inside the ASH, CT scans have been performed on an ASH unit operating at steady state to determine the time-averaged multiphase flow characteristics of ASH flotation. Figure 6 shows the multiphase flow characteristics inside an actual air-sparged hydrocyclone operating under industrial conditions as determined by X-ray CT. Details of the multiphase fluid flow have been established using X-ray CT analysis and the variation of the flow with operating conditions will be discussed in the following section.

3.1. Density Profiles

The essential feature of X-ray tomographic imaging is the determination of material density of a small region of three-dimensional space. Data obtained from the CT scanner are normally presented in an internationally standardized scale called the Hounsfield unit (CT number, which is determined by the attenuation coefficient discussed previously). To use the CT measurements for quantitative purposes, it is

Time-Averaged Density Profiles Inside ASH Using X-Ray CT

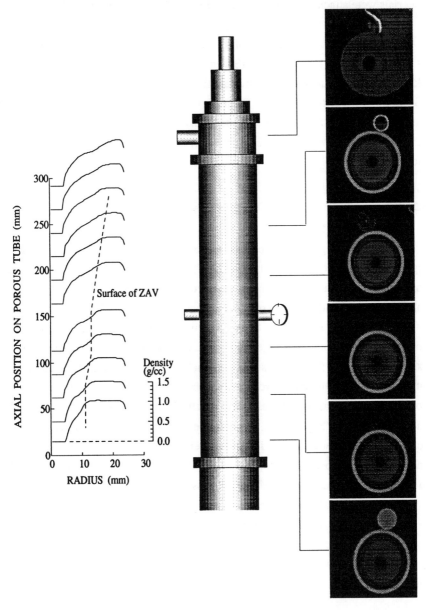

Fig. 6. Time-averaged density profiles during actual air-sparged hydrocyclone (ASH) flotation as determined by X-ray computed Tomography (CT).

necessary to do a calibration step with known density materials. As shown in th reconstructed tomographic images in the right-hand side of Fig. 6, several standar materials were attached on the exterior of the ASH unit for density calibration.

Figure 6 shows an example of the time averaged multiphase flow characteristi as revealed from CT data for an ASH unit treating a suspension of quartz particle (15% solids) with an amine collector at 12 psig inlet pressure and an air flow rate o 400 slpm. In the left-hand side of Figure 6, the time-average densities are plotted ver sus ASH radius for 11 different axial positions in the ASH. In addition, the surface o zero axial velocity (ZAV) obtained from tracer analysis is superimposed on the densit plot [10].

3.2. Characteristic Features of the Flow Regimes

By analyzing the scan sections made at different axial positions, information regarding the density profile (time-averaged) can be obtained for different operating conditions [10]. The flow regions as revealed by CT measurements for 5% and 15% solids in the feed and A* (ratio of overflow opening area to underflow opening area) = 1.0 are summarized in Figure 7. It can be seen that for 5% solids, the froth region does not extend to the bottom of the ASH unit. On the other hand, the froth region is extended for a 15% solids feed suggesting that froth phase stabilization increases with an increase in the amount of hydrophobic particles. The flotation recovery, i.e., transport of the hydrophobic particles to the overflow, is determined by the froth stability and the position of flow reversal. For both the conditions given in Figure 7, essentially complete flotation was achieved with recoveries of 94.2% and 97.2% for 5% solids and 15% solids respectively. However, when the conditions are changed and A* is set to 0.74, the froth phase decreases in thickness and extends the full length of the ASH. In this case, (A* = 0.74), the recovery of hydrophobic particles is reduced significantly to 68.4% as shown in Figure 8. On the basis of this quantitative x-ray CT analysis, conditions for effective flotation have been established and the effects of operating variables have been explained based on the characteristic features of the multiphase fluid flow [10].

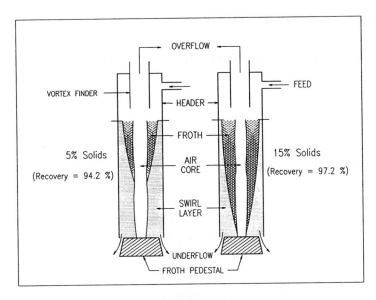

Fig. 7.   A comparison of the different froth features and flow regions with A*= 1.0, inlet pressure = 10.5 psi (slurry flow rate = 63 lpm) for 5% and 15% solids as determined by x-ray CT [10].

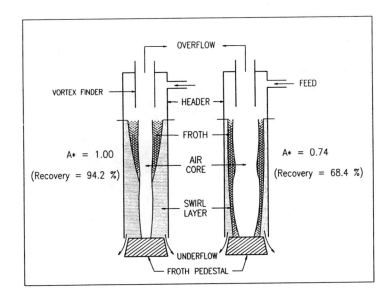

Fig. 8.   A comparison of different froth features and froth regimes with 5% solids in the feed, inlet pressure = 10.5 psi (slurry flow rate = 63 lpm) for two different values of A* as determined by x-ray CT [10].

4. On-Line Coal Washability Analysis

4.1. *Quantitative Coal Washability Analysis Using X-Ray CT*

Coal washability curves are important to the process engineer in the coal industry because it shows the limits for physical separation of mineral matter from coal. In fact, the washability curve provides information on the expected quality of the clean coal product.

Work done at the University of Utah indicates that X-ray CT can provide sufficient information to construct the washability curve within minutes of sample collection [11]. Figure 9 shows the schematic diagram for the measurement of a CT-based coal washability curve.

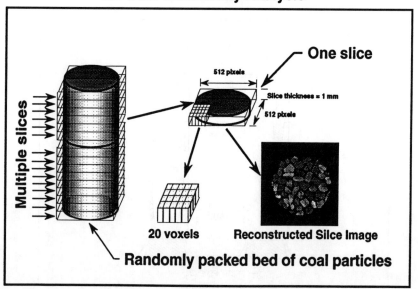

Schematic Diagram of a
Sequential X-Ray CT Scan of Coal Particles
for Coal Washability Analysis

Fig. 9.   Schematic diagram of sequential x-ray CT scan of coal samples for coal
washability analysis.

Figure 10 illustrates the washability curve for a coal sample as obtained by both the conventional sink-float analysis and the CT-based method. From these preliminary results, it is evident that coal washability curves derived from the CT-based technique are in good agreement with the results obtained by conventional sink-float analysis.

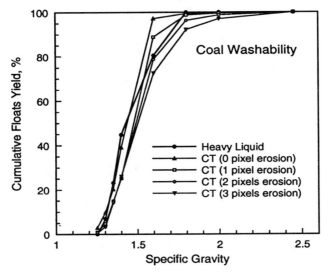

Fig. 10.   A comparison of the coal washability curve constructed using CT techniques with the coal washability curve obtained by the traditional sink-float method [11].

4.2.   CT-Based On-Line Coal Washability Analysis and Its Applications

In view of the success of laboratory studies using X-ray CT to determine coal washability and with the availability of high-speed CT systems, it now seems possible to design an on-line washability system for the control of coarse coal-cleaning circuits. Such a system would provide a new dimension to the operation of coal preparation plants. Figure 11 illustrates the proposed X-ray CT analyzer and sampling system for on-line coal washability analysis. Design features for such a system can be found in the literature [12].

There are many potential applications for an on-line washability analyzer. The feasibility of these applications is largely dependent on the system characteristics, i.e.

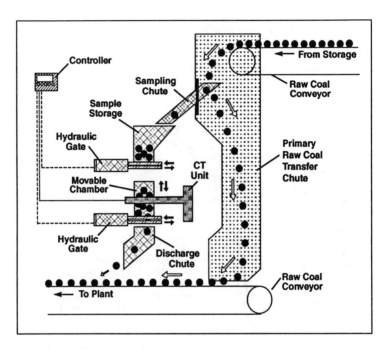

Fig. 11. A schematic view of the proposed X-ray CT analyzer and sampling system for on-line coal washability analysis [12].

accuracy, speed, and cost. Some of the most promising applications for the on-line CT system are variability analysis, blending control and on-line efficiency determination. Possible control strategies for these applications are described in the literature [12].

5. Conclusion

New algorithms have been developed to allow more accurate quantitative X-ray CT analysis for industrial applications. The effective use of quantitative X-ray CT techniques in the process engineering of particulate systems has been demonstrated. The time-averaged density profiles obtained from CT scans of an air-sparged hydrocyclone (ASH) flotation system operating in steady state have proved to be invaluable in helping to optimize design and operating variables. Furthermore, by using suitable algorithms, a CT-based method for the determination of coal-washability curves has been developed. The development of a CT analyzer for on-line coal washability is in progress and appears to have an excellent chance for successful implementation.

6. Acknowledgments

The authors wish to acknowledge the financial support from the Department of Energy, Grant No. DE-FG22-90PC90311, and the National Science Foundation, Grant No. CTS 9000406.

7. References

[1] G.T. Herman, Image Reconstruction from Projection: the Fundamentals of Computerized Tomography (Academic Press, New York, 1980), p. 316.

[2] W.F. Banholzer, et al., Ind. Eng. Chem. Res. 26 763-767 (1987).

[3] F. Natterer, Mathematics of Computerized Tomography (John Wiley & Sons, New York, 1986), p. 222.

[4] A.C. Kak and M. Slaney, Principles of Computerized Tomographic Imaging (IEEE Press, New York, 1988), p. 329.

[5] C.L. Lin, J.D. Miller, and A.B. Cortes, KONA 10 88-95 (1992).

[6] A.B. Cortes, C.L. Lin, and J.D. Miller, in Review of Progress in NDE, ed. D.O. Thompson and D.E. Chimenti, (Plenum Press, New York, 1985) pp. 459-467.

[7] J.D. Miller, et al., in Proceedings of XVI IMPC, ed. S.E. Forssberg (Elsevier, 1988) Part A, pp. 499-510.

[8] Y. Ye, et al., in Proceedings International Column Flotation Symposium, (AIME/SME, Phoenix, 1988), pp. 305-313.

[9] J.D. Miller and Y. Ye., J. of Mineral Processing and Extractive Metallurgy Review 5 307-329 (1989).

[10] J.D. Miller and A. Das., Minerals and Metallurgical Processing 12 51-63 (1995).

[11] C.L. Lin, et al., Int. J. of Coal Preparation 9 107-119 (1991).

[12] C.L. Lin, et al, in Proceedings High Efficiency Coal Preparation: An International Symposium, ed. S.K. Kawatra (AIME/SME, Denver, 1995), pp. 369-378.

Chapter 19

MRI for Assessing Mixing Quality

E.G. Smith[‡], R. Kohli[*], P. A. Martin[**], T. Instone[‡], N. Roberts[*], and R.H.T. Edwards[*]

‡ Unilever Research Port Sunlight Laboratory
Quarry Road East, Bebington, Wirral, L63 3JW, U.K.

* Magnetic Resonance Research Centre, University of Liverpool
PO Box 147, Liverpool, L69 3BX, U.K.

** General Electric Medical Systems (Europe)
78533 Buc Cedex, France

1. Introduction

Many of the crucial steps in the manufacture of consumer products such as detergents, personal products and foods, rely on the controlled mixing of ingredients to build in desirable heterogeneity. For example, the coexisting structures and properties of solid particles, emulsion droplets or liquid crystal phases and the diffusion of molecules between them often determine the stability, texture and performance characteristics of soap bars, powders, ice-cream, toothpaste, etc.. The manufacturing industry therefore has a fundamental interest in capturing knowledge of and monitoring, these processes at any stage.

Although by virtue of its sensitivity to molecular mobility and therefore physical state, NMR relaxation time spectroscopy has found widespread application in studies of phase composition and diffusion in these materials, the technique has necessarily been confined to average measurements on bulk samples. However, the recent extension of magnetic resonance imaging (MRI) [1] from medicine to industry has made it possible to examine some of these processes, spatially, in ways that are non-invasive and potentially quantitative [2, 3]. The attraction of MRI in process tomography resides in the fundamental relationships between NMR signal intensity and physical state, composition and molecular diffusion or flow. Numerous MRI applications have already been reported concerned with the visualization or spatial mapping of these properties in a variety of heterogeneous systems [4-8].

MRI is presently capable of achieving imaging times as short as 50-100msec. [9], spatial resolution of about 20μM [5] and measurement of components with T_2 relaxation times as low as 50μsec [10]. However, it is not usually possible to apply these specifications all at once and 'trade-offs' are necessary between imaging speed, scale and quantification, depending on the application involved and the equipment available. Although heterogeneity involving solid, semi-solid and liquid phases can be visualized quite satisfactorily with clinical whole-body systems, the limited RF and field gradient strengths restrict measurement of local signal intensity to components with relatively long T_2 relaxation times, (greater than a few milli-seconds).

In the spirit of advancing the concept of 'spatially determined NMR', the aim of this paper is to demonstrate some quantitative aspects of large-scale MRI on a whole-body imager in assessing mixing quality on model liquid systems. The emphasis is on the interpretation of image contrast in terms of local concentration and structure as a function of scale of scrutiny rather than on imaging speed.

Two model systems were chosen for our initial proton (^{1}H) MRI studies - one representing the case of non-interacting liquids mixing under laminar shear conditions and the other showing the formation of liquid crystal phases between surfactant and water. In the former case it was desirable to have a two component system, i.e., liquids A and B, with an exploitable difference in NMR relaxation time that could in principle represent a difference in their physical properties, e.g., viscosity, temperature, etc. An ideal choice was glycerine and paramagnetically doped (i.e., Cu^{2+} ions) glycerine undergoing shear in two mixing geometries - rotating concentric cylinders (Couette flow) and repetitive orifice flow. In the second case, the choice of materials was based on the known phase behavior of a commercial nonionic surfactant (alcohol ethoxylate) interacting with water to form liquid crystal structures [11], for which the NMR/MRI characteristics have already been established [12]. The model systems investigated, therefore, represent cases of distributive mixing and purely diffusive mixing of liquids.

2. Theory and principles

2.1 NMR Relaxation times (T_1 and T_2)

The T_1 (spin-lattice) and T_2 (spin-spin) relaxation times that govern longitudinal and transverse magnetization and therefore MRI signal intensity can be related to molecular mobility and hence to physical state as described by Bloembergen, Pound and Purcell [13]. These authors predict that, as mobility decreases, for liquids, T_1 and T_2 fall from, e.g., 2-3 seconds for pure water, to 10's of milliseconds for glycerine. In the case of restricted molecular mobility, as exists for liquid crystal chains, T_2 can be as low as 100μsec. T_2 for solids falls to 10's of μsec, with T_1 passing through a minimum where the frequency of motion corresponds to the NMR experimental frequency. T_1 and T_2 are also extremely sensitive to the presence of paramagnetic ions such as Cu^{2+}, Mn^{2+} or Gd^{3+} and this is often exploited in MRI to reduce T_1 for faster data acquisition or for improving contrast [14]. In the present study involving glycerine, aqueous $CuSO_4$ solution has been used to reduce T_2 of one of the components (B).

In the case of isotropic liquids, the T_2 relaxation curves are usually exponential in character and, for multi-component systems (A, B, C, etc.) the decay of intensity, I(t), follows the form :-

$$I(t) = I_A \exp\left[\frac{-t}{T_{2A}}\right] + I_B \exp\left[\frac{-t}{T_{2_B}}\right] + I_C \exp\left[\frac{-t}{T_{2C}}\right] \ldots \qquad \text{eq. (1).}$$

where I_A, I_B and I_C correspond to initial (t=0) signal intensities etc.

For an intimate molecular mixture where an average mobility or paramagnetic ion concentration and hence a single relaxation time (i.e., $\overline{T}_2$) can be assumed, the expression becomes :-

$$I = \left(I_A + I_B + I_C\right)\exp\left[\frac{-t}{\overline{T}_2}\right] \qquad \text{eq. (2).}$$

2.2 Quality of mixing

The quality of mixing is a subjective term and its assessment depends on the scale of scrutiny involved. Not surprisingly therefore, no standard definition of mixing quality has emerged that can be applied to every mixing scenario. Perhaps the most acceptable notion of 'thorough mixing' is one in which volumes of different materials are mixed until their individual building blocks are randomly distributed. The inevitable result of stirring or mixing two stable liquids under laminar shear conditions is the formation of striations that become thinner as more work is done on the system. This is equivalent to increasing interfacial area which in turn facilitates progress towards ultimate mixing via molecular diffusion between striations. The ultimate mixed state in the case of two miscible liquids, therefore, will be an inter-molecular blend possessing average liquid properties, e.g., viscosity, refractive index, etc. The above principles are covered in more detail elsewhere [15]. For components that interact to form new phases such as surfactant - water liquid crystals or precipitates, the quality of mixing observed is harder to define and depends on the nature of the molecular aggregates and the dynamics of their formation.

2.3 Partial Voluming

This effect occurs when image voxels contain only a part of the structures of interest and can lead to ambiguity in the information extracted from the images [16]. On the SIGNA system (GE Medical Systems, Milwaukee, WI) the lower limit on the pixel size, p, is fixed by the minimum field of view (FOV) of 8cm. and the image matrix of 512x512, i.e., $p = 150\mu M$. In the present studies, the FOV was fixed at 24cm and the image acquisition matrix was either 256x256 or 512x512, corresponding to $p = 940\mu M$ or $470\mu M$, respectively. With the striation thickness denoted by s, three cases can be considered:-

(i) *p >> s*   - here the pixel intensity, I, is determined by the relative intensities, I_A and I_B of liquid domains A and B in the voxel. Taking into account T_1 and T_2 relaxation after the repetition time, TR, and echo time, TE, respectively, (see sec. 3), I follows the form:-

$$I = I_A\left[1 - \exp\left(\frac{-TR}{T_{1A}}\right)\right]\exp\left(\frac{-TE}{T_{2_A}}\right) + I_B\left[1 - \exp\left(\frac{-TR}{T_{1_B}}\right)\right]\exp\left(\frac{-TE}{T_{2_B}}\right) \qquad \text{eq. (3).}$$

(ii) *p << s*   - in this case the two values of I would be resolvable across the image, corresponding to pure A and B components (as separate terms of equation 3).

(iii) *p ~ s* (*and molecular mixing*)   - in intermediate situations, a distribution of intensities is expected ranging between I_A and I_B. In the case of diffusion mixing where A and B are inter-molecularly mixed in a voxel, average values (i.e. $\overline{T}_1$ and $\overline{T}_2$) are assumed and the pixel intensity, I, becomes:-

$$I = (I_A + I_B)\left[1 - \exp\left(\frac{-TR}{\overline{T}_1}\right)\right]\exp\left(\frac{-TE}{\overline{T}_2}\right) \qquad \text{eq. (4).}$$

3. Methodology

3.1 MRI system and conditions

MRI data were obtained on a 1.5T GE SIGNA whole-body scanner using either a fast GRASS [17] or a spin-echo MRI sequence (TR= 200ms; TE = 20ms). The latter sequence was also used to measure T_2s on calibration samples. T_1 was measured by varying TR in suitable steps and by fixing TE.

3.2 Description of mixing systems and apparatus

Repetitive orifice flow - This term is used to describe a process where two liquids, in this case doped (B) and undoped (A) glycerine, are mixed by subjecting them to repeated flow through a constriction. With reference to Fig. 1a, a close fitting cylinder (top chamber) containing A is forced up and down into a second chamber containing B. The mixing occurs by deformation as the mixture passes through the hole or holes (ball-valve arrangement as in Fig. 1b) in the base of the upper cylinder and is aided by the reorientation of the striation in the downstream expansion zone.

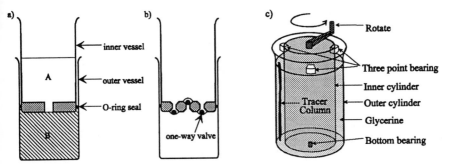

Fig. 1: Schematic of mixing apparatus used for MRI:- a) single orifice mixer; b) multi-orifice mixer; c) rotating cylinder system. Outer cylinder diameter = 14cm.

Laminar shear mixing (Couette flow) - the adoption of this system was inspired by the classic demonstration of reversibility of flow field of a Newtonian liquid such as glycerine between coaxial cylinders [Fig. 1c] in which a dyed tracer column is sheared and made to disappear by rotating the inner drum. If the direction of rotation is subsequently reversed, the tracer can be made to reappear quite spectacularly [see Fig. 6d]. There are several features that make this arrangement suitable for MRI studies of mixing. Firstly, the action is more relevant to industrial mixing situations. Secondly, the laminar shear conditions enable uniform striations of controllable thickness and composition to be examined. Finally, from an MRI point of view, the cylindrical symmetry eliminates the impact of the third dimension, so that a large slice thickness (i.e., d = 8mm) can be employed with obvious advantages in signal-to-noise ratio.

3.3 Choice of liquids and their calibration for MRI

Glycerine - was chosen for several reasons. Firstly, its high viscosity enables quantitative MRI pulse sequences to be explored within laminar flow regimes. Secondly, its miscibility with water allows stable layers of liquid to be set up containing different amounts of paramagnetic doping. Finally, since only small amounts of aqueous $CuSO_4$ solution (0.5% in glycerine) are used to produce the desired contrast, local image intensities are determined by variations in T_1 and T_2 and not by proton density.

The dependence of T_2 on percentage of doping (as a percentage of B in A, where B contains 4×10^{-3} moles of $CuSO_4$ in water) and the corresponding dependence of signal intensity on concentration for different values of TE are presented in Fig. 2. The curve for the shortest value of TE = 20ms was used in the interpretation of MRI data for mixing, using identical conditions on the scanner.

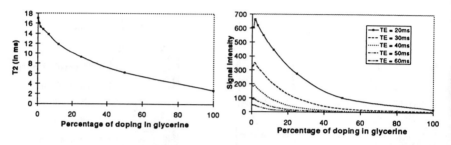

Fig. 2: NMR data for calibration samples

Surfactant-water - The nonionic surfactant (NI) used was commercial Dobanol 1-7 (Shell Chemicals (UK), Ltd.) which has an alkyl chain length of C_{11}, with an average of 7 moles of ethylene oxide per molecule comprising the head group.

4. Results and discussion

4.1 Repetitive orifice flow

In the first set of experiments, a T_2-weighted Fast GRASS MRI sequence (imaging time of 1 sec) was applied to the single orifice mixer to explore the nature of the mixing patterns developed between chambers in real time during 5 mixing cycles. A sequence of the images obtained is shown in Fig. 3 and the results are a clear demonstration of the ability of MRI to follow mixing effects between two liquids of differing NMR characteristics. However, the image contrast obtained, also highlights some of the current disadvantages of fast MRI sequences, e.g., in jeopardizing quantification for imaging speed. For instance, on the basis of the T_2 difference between doped and undoped glycerine the initial liquid in the bottom chamber should appear darker than that in the top chamber. The fact that this is not so is possibly due to the competing roles of T_1 and T_2 in determining the signal intensity under conditions of $T_1 > TR$, where the same value of I can be satisfied by different T_2 or T_1 values (or doping levels) [see eq. (3).] and even reversal of contrast is possible.

In Fig. 4, the mixing data obtained under quantitative MRI conditions using the spin echo sequence with long TR time (i.e., the T_1 term in eq. (3) becomes equal to 1) are compared for the two orifice geometries described. In both cases, the image contrast observed between the bottom and top chamber is in accord with the signal intensity versus concentration relationship of Fig. 2 and intermediate intensities obtained as mixing proceeds depend on the composition of a voxel as determined by partial volume effects or inter-molecular mixing. Since the imaging time was about 50sec, the mixing action had to be stopped during each data acquisition. Nevertheless, the rheological properties of the liquid used allowed the process of laminar flow to be interrupted without significant movement of the liquid during the imaging period.

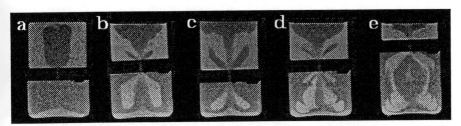

Fig. 3: Real time axial MR images (Fast GRASS) through single orifice mixer. a) ¼ displacement (down); b) 1 complete cycle (down-up top-down centre); c) 3 cycles; d) 5 cycles; e) 5½ cycle.

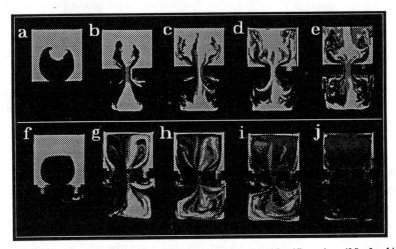

Fig. 4: MR spin echo images of a single orifice mixer (a-e) and multi-orifice mixer (f-j) after ¼, 1, 2, 3, and 5 cycles.

Using the method of pixel counting, the data were analyzed to produce 'histograms' of MR intensity distribution across the images as in Fig. 5, where the heights of the columns represent the normalized pixel counts for the intensity bands (related to the liquid composition) indicated on the horizontal axis. As expected, the first histogram in the series shows mainly two peaks corresponding to doped (B) and undoped or pure liquid (A). As mixing proceeds, an increase in the percentage of intermediate regions at the expense of the unmixed ones is clearly demonstrated. The same trend is also observed for the multi-orifice mixer although this occurs at a much faster rate. In the latter configuration the ball-valve system (Fig. 1b) promotes circulation of the liquid up through the central hole and down through the outer holes with a similar action to that of some commercial non-intrusive mixers.

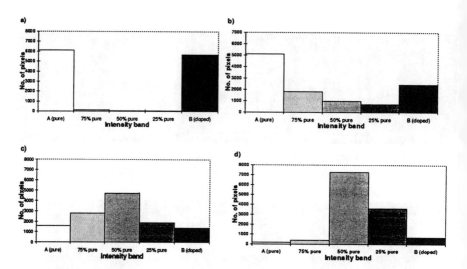

Figure 5: MRI intensity histograms (pixel counts for each intensity or voxel composition.) a) zero mixing; b) 3 cycles with single orifice; c) 3 cycles with multi-orifice; d) 5 cycles with multi-orifice.

In contrast to single orifice mixing, the state of mixing reached by the multi-hole system indicates an almost uniform distribution of intensities after only three cycles. The final histogram shows almost complete disappearance of the outer peaks, suggesting inter-molecular mixing. However, a high mid peak is not a sufficient condition of inter-molecular mixing since partial voluming can produce a similar effect at thinner striations. The state of complete mixing can only be achieved via the process of molecular diffusion, which in the case of glycerine, is slow. Nevertheless, when the striation thickness, s, reduces below about 400μM, intermolecular diffusion can become significant over the time scale of the mixing experiment.

4.2 Laminar shear mixing

Fig. 6 and 7 compare the results of laminar shear mixing for two different experiments using the apparatus of Fig. 1c - (i) a three column (doped glycerine) method [Fig. 6] and (ii) an arrangement in which the coaxial space (1.5cm) is divided vertically and equally between doped and undoped glycerine [Fig. 7b]. The advantage of the latter method over the tracer method is that the rotation of the inner drum produces light and dark striations of similar thickness that become thinner as the mixing proceeds. The ability of the technique to image any plane through the object is demonstrated in the pictures of Fig. 7a and 7b.

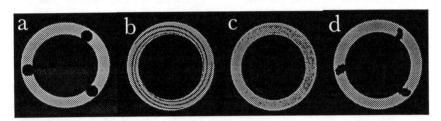

Figure 6: MRI coronal sections through rotation apparatus (3 tracer experiment) showing 'reversibility' of flow or the 'unmixing' effect. a) initial set-up; b) after 1 turn clockwise; c) further 19 turns clockwise; d) after 20 turns anti-clockwise.

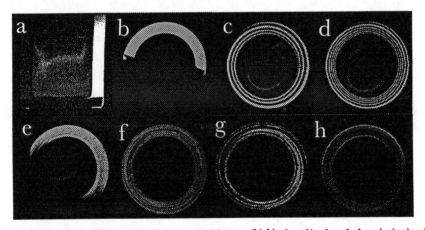

Figure 7: MRI results using equally divided co-axial space (½,½, doped/undoped glycerine). a) axial image through apparatus; b-h) coronal images: b) at t = 0; c) after 3 turns clockwise; d) a further 2 turns; e) after reversing 5 turns; f) new experiment; after 20 turns clockwise; g) followed by reversal (20 turns); h) new experiment - 20 clockwise turns, wait 30 mins, then reverse 20 turns.

Assuming the cross-sectional area, A, of doped glycerine remains constant during shear, the striation thickness, s, is estimated to range from about 10μM to 2mm (using the simple relation :- $A \sim 2\pi Rsn$; where n is the number of revolutions and R is the mean coaxial radius; 6.5cm). The effect of pixel size on image resolution is apparent when striations are at their thinnest, i.e., as shown in Fig. 6c and 7f.

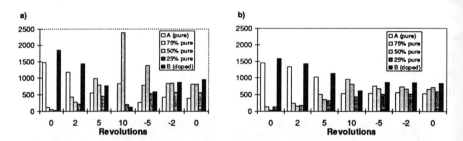

Fig. 8: MR intensity histograms for two imaging resolutions, a) 256x256 and, b) 512x512.

Partial voluming effects and possible diffusion mixing can be explored using two different pixel sizes. Comparing the histograms of Fig. 8a and 8b, the initial states (0 revolutions) are similar, as expected from such large cross-sections of doped and undoped regions (outer peaks) compared to the pixel size. Only after two or more revolutions are differences apparent. For 10 revolutions, where the striation thickness is about 750µM, a 256 X 256 image (p = 940µM) indicates almost complete absence of the outer peaks in favor of a peak in the intermediate region (Fig. 8a), which could be interpreted as inter-molecular mixing. However, the equivalent histogram for the higher resolution image (i.e., 512 X 512, p = 470µM) indicates the survival of 'pure' (white) and doped (black) striations over the rotations (Fig. 8b). This striation integrity is supported by the reappearance of the outer peaks in the lower resolution experiment upon reversing the direction of rotation. This would certainly not be allowed if intermolecular mixing via random molecular diffusion was complete. Conversely, the survival of intermediate peaks after reversal (-10 revolutions), shown in Fig. 8a and 8b can be taken as an indication of some diffusive mixing.

D_{self} for glycerine is relatively low, i.e., 2.5 x 10^{-8} cm^2.sec^{-1} [18]. Hence, the mean displacement, x, of a molecule during time, Δt = 30mins, due to diffusion, as expected from the Einstein relation [19] i.e., :- $\langle x^2 \rangle = 6D_{self}\Delta t$ is about 150µM. That molecular diffusion over this distance can have an effect on the mixing is demonstrated by the results of a 20 revolution experiment in which the reversibility with and without a 30min waiting time between the rotation directions is compared (Fig. 7g and 7h). Although not shown here, the corresponding histograms indicate a displacement of peaks towards the lower intensity bands (doped end) upon diffusion, i.e., suggestive of signal intensity values controlled by molecularly mixed rather than partially volumed composition within a voxel (compare I for eq. (3) and (4)). This same effect can be seen in the data for the multi-orifice mixing. (Fig. 5d).

4.3 Diffusive mixing of surfactant-water

This section examines briefly the potential of MRI in mixing of more complex components, in particular those capable of forming new phases when molecularly mixed. The example is taken from other NMR work [12] concerned with the phase behavior of nonionic surfactant (Dobanol 1-7) with water and has relevance in the processing, storage and use of products containing these components.

Fig. 9 shows the interaction between nonionic surfactant (NI) and water using similar MRI sequences to those described in section 3.1. In contrast to the glycerine experiments, no paramagnetic doping is applied and yet a range of image contrast is developed over time, indicating that structural changes accompanying molecular diffusion have occurred.

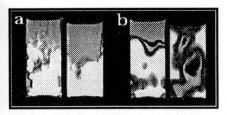 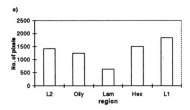

Figure 9: Axial spin echo MR images through tubes containing nonionic surfactant, NI, and water (H_2O). a) left-hand image- water poured over NI; right-hand image- NI poured over water. b) as for a), but after 3 days; c) MR intensity histogram representing spatial phase analysis of NI/water mixture.

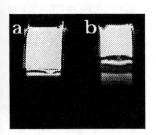 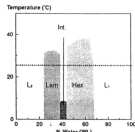

Figure 10: a) MR image of NI layer on D_2O layer after time $t \sim 0$; b) after 8 days; c) phase map for Dobanol 1-7 nonionic surfactant and water.

Equilibrium phase diagrams (Fig. 10c) established from a range of complementary techniques, e.g., x-ray, NMR and microscopy, indicate that for this system, two structured liquid crystal (LC) phases are formed over the composition range namely, hexagonal (Hex) and lamellar (Lam), in which surfactant molecules agglomerate, respectively, into regular rod-like and sandwich-like structures separated by water [11]. In addition to nonionic-rich (L_2) and water-rich (L_1) solution phases, there is also a region of oily liquid between the LC phases. The surfactant chains in LC configurations possess lower mobility than liquid phases and the corresponding (^{1}H) T_2 values (100-200μsec) lead to lower intensities in the MR images [12].

The effects observed in the experiments of Fig. 9a and 9b can be interpreted with the aid of MR images obtained for diffusive mixing between adjacent layers of surfactant and deuterium oxide (D_2O) (- used to avoid water signal). In Fig. 10b the light and dark bands produced as diffusion occurs between the components can be assigned, with reference to the phase diagram, to alternate layers of liquid and LC phases appropriate to the concentration gradient developed down the sample tube. An analogous calibration approach to that used in the glycerine system, involving T_1 and T_2 measurements on pure phases was used in the analysis. By means of unique T_1 and T_2 relationships determined for each phase, the relative composition can be identified from the T_1 and T_2 weighted images. An example of the composition histograms for the mixed system is shown in Fig. 9c.

5. Conclusions and prospects

These exploratory MRI studies have helped to identify some of the key requirements for quantitative MR tomography of mixing processes using a conventional whole-body scanner. Because of current limitations on imaging speed and short T_2 measurements, the initial emphasis has been on mapping of composition, or structure, in non-interacting and phase-forming liquids.

The results have demonstrated how relaxation time NMR of the type used to analyze phase composition can be extended to spatial studies of dynamic heterogeneity in industrially relevant systems. In the assessment of mixing quality, the virtues of an NMR-based tomography make it worthwhile in future to extend the level of scrutiny to the determination of the level of inter-molecular mixing within a voxel by means of, for example, T_2 decay analysis.

The MRI observation of the phases formed between surfactant and water in real-time under non-equilibrium conditions are, we believe, the first of their kind, and the results have implications for MR tomography applications on other interacting multi-component system. The most obvious future requirement for quantitative MR process tomography is the bringing together of developments in rapid imaging, high spatial resolution and short-T_2 capability.

6. Acknowledgements
The authors acknowledge Dr. R. B. Edwards for helpful discussions.

7. References

[1] P. C. Lauterbur, Nature. **242**: pp.190-191, (1973)

[2] P. Mansfield and P. G. Morris, <u>NMR Imaging in Biomedicine</u>, Adv. Magn. Reson. Supp2. New York, Academic Press, (1982)

[3] B. Blumich and W. Kuhn, <u>Magnetic Resonance Microscopy</u> (Methods and Applications in Materials Science, Agriculture and Bio-medicine), VCH, New York, (1992)

[4] E. G. Smith, J. W. Rockliffe, P. J. McDonald, A. Lonagan, M. R Halse, B. Leone and J. H. Strange, Magn. Reson. Imaging, Vol. 12, No. 2, pp231-234, (1994)

[5] C. J. Rofe, R. K. Lambert and P. T. Callaghan, J. Rheol., **38**, (4), July, pp875-887, (1994)

[6] R. J. Phillips, AICHE Symposium Series, **89**, (1993)

[7] L. D. Hall, V. Rajanayagam and C. Hall, J. Magn. Reson., **68**, p185, (1986)

[8] J. B. German and M. J. McCarthy, J. Agric. Food Chem., **37**, pp1321-1324, (1989)

[9] P. Mansfield, J. Phys. C. **10**, L55 (1977)

[10] K. L. Perry, P. J. McDonald, E. W. Randall and K. Zick, Polymer, **35**, p2744, (1994)

[11] D. J. Mitchell, G. J. T. Tiddy, L. Waring, T. Bostock and M. P. McDonald, J. Chem. Soc. Faraday. Trans 1, **79**, pp975-1000, (1983)

[12] E. G. Smith, T. Instone, J. W. Rockliffe and L. Kelly, (unpublished work)

[13] N. Bloembergen, E. M. Purcell and R. V. Pound, Phys. Rev., **73**, p679, (1948)

[14] M. Graif, G. M. Bydder and R. E. Steiner, AGNR, **6**, pp855-862, (1985)

[15] N. Harnby, M. F. Edwards and A. W. Nienow, <u>Mixing in the Process Industry</u>, Butterworths, pp1-7 and pp202-225, (1985)

[16] N. Roberts, G. Nesbitt and T. Fenz, Nondestr. Test. Eval., **11**, pp273-291, (1994)

[17] A. Haase, J. Frahm, D. Matthaei, W. Hanicke and K. D. Merboldt, J. Magn. Reson., **67**, pp258-266, (1986)

[18] E. O. Stejskal and J. E. Tanner, J. Chem. Phys., **42**, p288, (1965)

[19] A. Einstein, <u>Investigations in the Theory of Brownian Movement</u>, Dover, New York, (1956)

Chapter 20

Tracking Positron-emitting Tracers in Industrial Processes

D J Parker, D M Benton, P Fowles, P A McNeil and Min Tan
University of Birmingham Positron Imaging Centre
School of Physics and Space Research, The University of Birmingham
Birmingham B15 2TT UK

. Introduction

The use of radioactive tracers offers unrivalled possibilities for the study of industrial processes, but also suffers from some restrictions. Gamma-rays can penetrate a considerable thickness of metal, enabling imaging to be carried out on real plant, and very small quantities of tracer can be detected, so that an individual component of a multi-phase flow system can be labelled and its behaviour observed. However, detection involves the counting of individual γ-ray photons, which is generally slow, and the need to avoid release of radioactivity means that tracers are best used in closed systems.

Some examples of process studies using γ-ray emission imaging have been reported and were recently reviewed [1]. Although several approaches to the tomographic imaging of radioactive tracers are well established in medicine, it appears that the only one which has made much impact in engineering studies is the use of positron-emitting tracers. The positron, being the anti-particle of the normal electron, rapidly annihilates with an electron and their combined energy is released in the form of a pair of 511keV γ-rays which are emitted back-to-back, 180° apart, in order to conserve momentum. Thus simultaneous detection of these two γ-rays on either side of the system defines a line passing through the point of emission, and by measuring the number of such "events" detectable along each line of sight a tomographic image of the tracer distribution can be obtained.

Positron emission tomography (PET) is increasingly being used in medicine fo[...] studying organ function [2], but medical PET scanners designed to accomodate [...] human body are often not convenient for industrial imaging. At Birmingham, [...] "positron camera" [3] designed for engineering studies has been in use since 1984 [4] This chapter briefly summarizes the principal ways in which it has been operated an[...] the applications which have been studied. As an alternative to imaging of fluid tracers a method for tracking a single labelled particle has been developed and is proving very powerful.

2. Principles of positron-based imaging

2.1 *Positron-emitting Tracers*

One of the ways in which a nuclide with an excess of protons in the nucleu[...] can become more stable is to undergo positive β-decay, in which a proton is converted into a neutron with emission of a positron. Such nuclides are generally produced in nuclear reactions using particle accelerators such as cyclotrons. Most are very short lived, but some have half-lives of days or even years. The tracers most commonly used in medical PET, with their half-lives, are ^{11}C (20 mins), ^{13}N (10 mins), ^{15}O (2 mins) and ^{18}F (110 mins); these can be synthesized into organic molecules prior to injection into the body. For non-medical imaging the requirements are different, and it is generally convenient to use a tracer with a longer half-life: those used at Birmingham to date include ^{68}Ga (68 mins), ^{18}F (110 mins), ^{61}Cu (3.4 hours), ^{64}Cu (12.7 hours), ^{140}Nd (3.4 days) and ^{22}Na (2.6 years). All these nuclides are cyclotron produced, apart from ^{68}Ga and ^{64}Cu. ^{64}Cu can be produced using a cyclotron, but is more easily obtained by exposing copper to thermal neutrons from a nuclear reactor. ^{68}Ga is the daughter of ^{68}Ge (half-life 288 days) and can be eluted in solution from a "generator" containing the long-lived parent, providing a convenient portable source of short-lived tracer.

Tracers are used either in solution or as small particles. For fluid imaging the usual requirement is that the tracer follows the component of interest and does not react with other components present. Cation tracers are convenient in that they can be complexed to give appropriate behaviour - complexing with EDTA creates a chemically-inert form which is soluble in aqueous solution, while complexing with a chelating agent produces an organically-soluble form. Solid tracer particles are currently made by irradiating glass beads or sand on a cyclotron so as to generate ^{18}F from the oxygen content; sufficient activity for single particle tracking can be generated in a 1mm diameter particle, and techniques for labelling smaller particles are being developed.

The emitted positron rapidly slows down in matter and comes to rest before annihilating with an electron. From a given nuclide, positrons are emitted with a continuous range of energies extending up to the maximum determined by the difference in mass between initial and final states. For most of the tracers listed above, this maximum energy is between 1 and 2 MeV, corresponding to a maximum distance travelled by the positron of between 2 and 4 mm in aluminium. However, in general the distance between the point of emission and the point at which annihilation occurs is much less than this because (i) the emitted positron typically has significantly less energy than the maximum possible, and (ii) the positron does not travel in a straight line. The distance travelled is inversely proportional to the density of the medium, so it is clear that using the γ-rays arising from annihilation to determine the location of the emitting tracer is reasonable in any solid or liquid medium but not in a gas.

Annihilation of the positron with an electron gives rise to a pair of 511 keV γ-rays which are emitted 180° apart to within 0.1°. These γ-rays are quite penetrating; 50% emerge unscattered after traversing 3 cm Al or 1.1 cm Fe, implying the possibility of imaging through standard engineering casings. However, the remainder are mostly scattered, and can give rise to a background in the data. For some nuclides, background also arises from other γ-rays which accompany the decay process; of the list above, this affects only ^{61}Cu and ^{22}Na.

2.2 Positron-based imaging at Birmingham

Unlike most medical PET systems, which consist of one or more rings of scintillator detectors, the Birmingham positron camera [3] shown in Fig. 1 consists of two gas-filled chambers which are placed either side of the volume to be imaged. Each has an active area 60 x 30 cm^2; a γ-ray interacting within this area can be located to within about 8 mm, but unfortunately only about 7% of the γ-rays incident on each detector are detected. Only coincidence events in which γ-rays are detected in both detectors "simultaneously" (i.e. within 25 ns) are processed, their coordinates being stored event-by-event on computer, together with the time of arrival, for subsequent processing. The combination of the poor detection efficiency and the need to avoid excessive rates of random coincidences limits the maximum useful counting rate of the camera to around 3000 coincidence events per second. The mount shown in Fig. 1 enables the separation and alignment of the detectors to be varied to suit the application [4]. The camera is used in three distinct ways: for 2D projection imaging or 3D tomographic imaging of a fluid tracer, or for tracking of a single tracer particle.

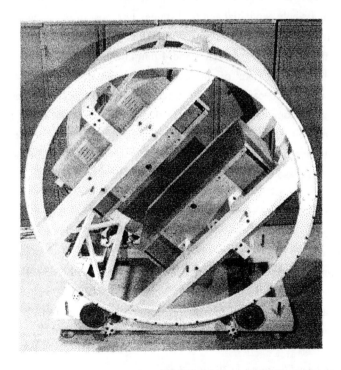

Fig. 1: The two detectors of the Birmingham positron camera on their rotating mount.

With the detectors stationary and well-separated, a single 2D projected view of the distribution of a fluid tracer parallel to the detector faces is obtained, which is particularly useful if the tracer is known to be confined to a relatively narrow band in the orthogonal direction. An image can be obtained in around 60s, with a spatial resolution of 8mm (full-width at half maximum of the point spread function).

Although such a projection image is not tomographic, it can in principle be made fully quantitative, unlike in some other imaging modalities. Correction must be made for the attenuation of the γ-rays emitted along each observed line of sight, but this is straightforward since the probability of removal of one or other of the pair of back-to-back γ-rays is just given by the total amount of attenuating material on their path, independent of where along this path the annihilation occurred. The attenuation can if necessary be measured for each line of sight using an external source. Some examples of 2D projection imaging of a bolus of tracer are given in the next section.

To obtain a 3D tomographic image of the tracer distribution, the detectors must be rotated through 180° about the field of view so as to measure projected views at all angles. The mount shown in Fig. 1 rocks backwards and forwards, taking approximately 45 s for each 180° scan, during which data is recorded continuously. Images are reconstructed by backprojection into a 3D array of voxels, and are quantitative provided attenuation corrections are made as described above. The intrinsic spatial resolution is 8mm in each coordinate, but in practice images are often limited by noise due to poor counting statistics, so that it is necessary to introduce further smoothing. Around an hour is required to obtain enough data to reconstruct a reasonable 3D image of an extended tracer distribution, so that the principal application for this technique is the imaging of steady-state distributions. For example, the first use of the positron camera was for observing the lubricant distribution within operating aero-engines and gearboxes [5]. The next chapter describes another application, where PET has been used to image the distribution of individual size fractions of the sand within a stirred slurry by selectively labelling a selected size fraction.

For dynamic studies, the technique of Positron Emission Particle Tracking (PEPT) has been developed at Birmingham [6]. Instead of using a fluid tracer whose distribution is imaged, in PEPT a single labelled tracer particle is introduced into the system under study and is tracked in 3D. The tracer location can be determined by triangulation using a sample containing only a small number of detected pairs of back-to-back γ-rays, and so can be obtained many times per second. For a moving tracer there is an optimum sample size, such that the statistics are adequate but the tracer does not move too far during location, and an algorithm has been developed which adjusts to the speed of the tracer so that as the speed increases the sample size decreases. PEPT is normally performed with the detectors separated by 30cm; in thi geometry a slow moving tracer particle can be located to within about 1mm in 3D 5 times per second and a particle moving at 1m/s to within 5mm 250 times per second Thus locations are not equally spaced in time, but the time corresponding to eacl location is accurately known from the recorded times of arrival of the γ-ray pairs used in its determination. By taking the difference between successive locations a measure of the instantaneous vector velocity of the tracer can also be obtained; with a certair amount of smoothing this is generally accurate to within 10% [4].

Some of the applications of the PEPT technique will be described in Section 4 below. In order to provide relevant information, the tracer particle must be isokinetic with the surrounding material; to date studies have concentrated on granular materials, where the motion of one particle is followed within a bed of many similar particles, but it is also possible to conceive of using a neutrally-buoyant tracer particle to study flow in a fluid. Because only a single tracer particle is tracked, it is easiest to obtain representative results in a closed recirculating system.

3. Applications of 2D projection imaging

As stated above, the Birmingham positron camera takes around a minute to measure a single 2D projection image - the more extended the tracer distribution, the longer it takes to obtain a good image. For this reason, the camera has mainly been used to study relatively slow flow processes, such as flow through geological materials. Fig. 2 shows a series of 10 minute images of the passage of a bolus of water containing the tracer ^{18}F through a sample of oil-reservoir sandstone ($5 \times 5 cm^2$, 30cm long) which was saturated with brine. In similar studies, the displacement of oil by brine has been observed, with either the oil phase or the aqueous phase being labelled. Uptake of water into dry porous stone or brick by capillary action is another area of current study. Extensive work has also been carried out on imaging flow through fractures in impermeable rock (slate or limestone), where the specimens were selected to have approximately planar fractures suitable for 2D imaging. After filling the fracture with non-sorbing tracer of known concentration the image provides the absolute fracture thickness at each point, while using a bolus of such tracer the flow streams can be studied. Sorbing tracers have also been investigated, and present work is mainly concerned with observing two-phase gas-liquid flow within a fracture.

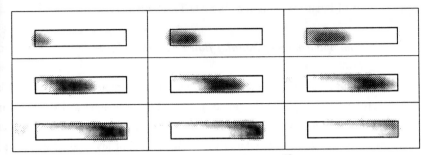

Fig. 2: Sequence of 2D projection images of a bolus of ^{18}F tracer in solution, passing through a 30cm long sample of porous sandstone. A 10 minute image was recorded every 30 minutes.

Attempts have also been made to apply the technique to studying the extrusion of pastes. Fig. 3 shows a sequence of images of a single line of labelled paste, initially 76mm long, which was laid down between layers of inactive paste in order to mark a flow front as the paste was extruded through a nozzle. In this case the extrusion was halted after every 40ml and an image was recorded with the paste stationary; each image is based on only 40,000 detected events, corresponding to approximately 15s data at the maximum useful rate. Although the images suffer from background due to noise, the flow front is sufficiently clear. However, 15s is still too long an imaging time for most extrusion processes.

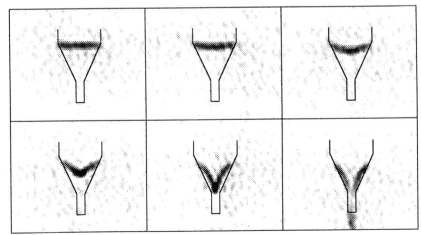

Fig. 3: Sequence of 2D projection images of a line of ^{68}Ga-labelled paste, initially 76mm long, during extrusion through a conical nozzle.

4. Applications of Positron Emission Particle Tracking

4.1 Example of an application - Granular flow in a rolling drum

Data from a study of granular flow and mixing in a simple rolling drum [7] is presented here as an example of the power of the PEPT technique and the ways in which the data can be analysed. A horizontal axis cylindrical drum, internal diameter 136mm, was filled to 32% of its volume with 1.5mm glass beads, one of which had been irradiated so that it contained ^{18}F and served as the tracer particle. The PEPT technique was used to track this tracer as the drum was rotated at 33 rpm about its axis. After processing, the data consist of a series of locations (x,y,z), each with its associated time (the interval between locations is not constant, but decreases as the tracer speed increases).

A qualititative impression of the behaviour can be obtained by replaying the tracer motion on a computer screen. Quantitative analysis generally involves integrating the behaviour over a long period, so as to obtain a representative sample of all the possible types of behaviour. Thus the grey scales in Fig. 4(a) show the fraction of time spent by the tracer at each point in the transaxial plane during a 2 hour run; assuming that the tracer behaviour is truly representative of all the other particles in the drum, this measures the number density of particles at each point. The arrows in Fig. 4(b) show the average in-plane velocity at each point. Two distinct regions are apparent: the lower part of the bed rotates with the drum while the upper part slides downwards. From these data, parameters such as the thickness of the sliding layer can easily be extracted. However, average values of velocity alone are insufficient to characterise the behaviour fully. Fig. 5 shows the distributions of velocity values observed within two small regions (one near the bottom of the bed, and the other in the sliding layer at the top) over the same 2 hour period. Much greater internal motion is seen within the sliding layer than in the lower part of the bed. All the data are of course three-dimensional, and the results could also be divided into separate axial slices, but in this particular study the behaviour is expected to be independent of axial position, and so all observations have been averaged over the length of the drum.

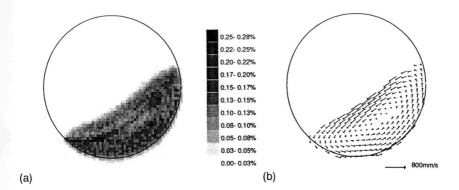

(a)   (b)

Fig. 4: (a) Fraction of total run time spent by the tracer particle at each transaxial position within the rolling drum (the plane has been divided into 2.5x2.5 mm^2 pixels). (b) Average velocity of the tracer particle at each transaxial position.

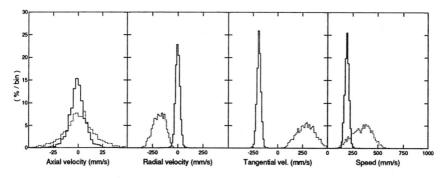

Fig. 5: Distributions of tracer particle velocities observed in two distinct 10x10 mm^2 transaxial regions within the rolling drum: near the bottom of the bed (solid) and in the sliding layer (dotted). Note the expanded scale used for the axial velocity component.

Such a rolling drum produces slow axial mixing. In order to quantify this, the axial displacement of the tracer from its initial position has been extracted as a function of time. Since mixing is expected to be independent of axial position, every observed tracer location has been taken as a valid starting point; the distributions in Fig. 6 show the subsequent axial deviation with time, and therefore correspond to the dispersion of an initially thin slice of particles. From such distributions, values such as mixing indices or diffusion coefficients can be extracted.

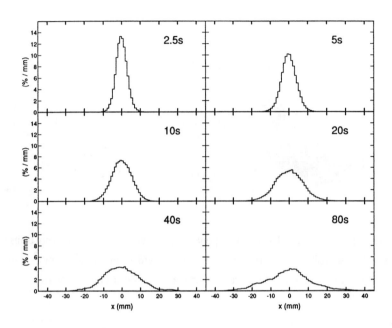

Fig. 6: Distributions showing the axial displacement of the tracer particle with time within the rolling drum.

4.2 Other PEPT applications

To date the PEPT technique has mainly been applied to studies of granular mixing, but fluidised beds are being increasingly studied, and investigations of hopper flow have also been made.

Most of the mixing studies have been carried out in small batch mixers containing blades. For example, studies have been made of the effect of blade speed [8] and fill level [9] on mixing in a 5 litre horizontal-axis ploughshare mixer, using analysis like that described above. An unexpected observation was that under many conditions the vessel separated into two well-mixed compartments axially, with material exchanging only occasionally between cells. In this case the PEPT results have also been used to determine the average residence time in each compartments, and the circumstances of transfer. Since information on shaft angle can be recorded at the same time as the positron camera data, the results can also be correlated with the position of the blades.

Initial studies of particle motion in a gas-fluidised bed have concentrated on measuring the circulation time [10] and characterising the sudden jumps associated with capture by a bubble [11]. From an initial study of hopper flow, carried out by emptying a cylindrical hopper containing a tracer particle 50 times, the variation in the velocity with radius and height above the orifice has been extracted and compared with kinematic theory [12].

5. Summary

This chapter has outlined some of the industrial applications of positron-based imaging tackled in Birmingham to date. The positron camera is capable of producing a 3D tomographic image with a spatial resolution of 8mm, but this requires a large volume of data which takes around an hour to measure, and so is principally useful for steady-state imaging; as described in the next chapter, this provides a unique way of observing segregation. A single 2D projection image can be obtained in around a minute, and flow studies involving the imaging of a slow moving bolus of tracer have proved useful in some situations. However, the most exciting use of the positron camera appears to be for single particle tracking, since a tracer particle moving at 1m/s can be located in 3D to within 5mm approximately 250 times per second, and its velocity determined each time to within 10%. In the previous section, some of the ways in which such data can be used to investigate processes such as mixing were discussed. The technique is most useful for closed systems where a single tracer particle eventually maps out all the possible types of behaviour.

Some of the limitations of the present positron camera could be overcome with improved technology. In particular, a hybrid design of positron camera has recently developed which offers the possibility of at least a tenfold increase in data rates [13]. The estimated cost of such a system is around £0.5M; this cost, together with the complications involved in using radioactive tracers, suggests that positron-based imaging will continue to be used only as a research tool for studying the behaviour of model plant, rather than for on-line monitoring. Nevertheless it is possible to conceive the development of much simpler on-line systems giving poorer spatial resolution and used in conjunction with a short-lived positron-emitter such as ^{82}Rb (half-life 1.3 min), which is obtainable from a generator containing its parent ^{82}Sr (25 days).

6. References

[1]   D.J. Parker, M.R. Hawkesworth and T.D. Beynon, Chemical Eng. Journal **56** 109-117 (1995)

[2]   S.M. Tilyou, J. Nucl. Med. **32** 15N-26N (1991)

[3]   M.R. Hawkesworth, M.A. O'Dwyer, J. Walker, P. Fowles, J. Heritage, P.A.E. Stewart, R.C. Witcomb, J.E. Bateman, J.F. Connolly and R. Stephenson, Nucl. Instr. & Methods **A253** 145-157 (1986)

[4]   D.J. Parker, M.R. Hawkesworth, C.J. Broadbent, P. Fowles, T.D. Fryer and P.A. McNeil, Nucl. Instr. & Methods **A348** 583-592 (1994)

[5]   P.A.E. Stewart, J.D. Rogers, R.T. Skelton, P.L.Salter, M.J. Allen, R. Parker, P. Davis, P. Fowles, M.R. Hawkesworth, M.A. O'Dwyer, J. Walker and R. Stephenson, in Non-destructive Testing, Proc. 4th Eur. Conf., London 1987, ed. J.M. Farley and R.W. Nichols (Pergamon, Oxford, 1988) pp 2718-2726

[6]   D.J. Parker, C.J. Broadbent, P. Fowles, M.R. Hawkesworth and P.A. McNeil, Nucl. Instr. & Methods **A326** 592-607 (1993)

[7]   D.J. Parker, A.E. Dijkstra and P.A. McNeil, in Proceedings of ECAPT'95, ed. M.S. Beck et al. (UMIST, Manchester, 1995) pp 352-360

[8]   J. Bridgwater, C.J. Broadbent and D.J. Parker, Trans. I. Chem. E **71A** 675-681 (1993)

[9]   C.J. Broadbent, J. Bridgwater and D.J. Parker, Chemical Eng. Journal **56** 119-125

[10]   J.P.K. Seville, S.J.R. Simons, C.J. Broadbent, D.J. Parker and T.D. Beynon, in Proceedings of 1st Int. Particle Tech. Forum, Denver (AIChE, 1994) **I** pp 493-498

[11]   J.P.K. Seville, S.J.R. Simons, C.J. Broadbent, T.W. Martin, D.J. Parker and T.D. Beynon, in Proceedings of Fluidization VIII (Engineering Foundation, 1995) to be published

[12]   J.P.K. Seville, T.W. Martin and D.J. Parker, in Proceedings of 3rd European Symposium on Storage and Flow of Particulate Solids, Nurnberg, 1995, to be published

[13]   K. Wells, D. Visvikis, R.J. Ott, J.E. Bateman, R. Stephenson, J. Connolly and G. Tappern, Nucl. Instr. and Methods **A348** 600-606 (1994)

Chapter 21

VISUALIZATION OF SIZE-DEPENDENT PARTICLE SEGREGATION IN SLURRY MIXERS USING POSITRON EMISSION TOMOGRAPHY

S. L. McKee
Satake Centre for Grain Process Engineering
Dept. of Chemical Engineering
University of Manchester Institute of Science and Technology
Manchester M60 1QD, UK

D. J. Parker
Positron Imaging Centre
School of Physics and Space Research
University of Birmingham
Edgbaston, Birmingham, B15 2TT, UK

R. A. Williams
Particle & Colloid Engineering Group
Camborne School of Mines
University of Exeter
Redruth
Cornwall, TR15 3SE, UK

1.0 Introduction

The operation of mixing solid particles in a liquid is encountered in a variety of chemical processes including dissolution, crystallization and mass transfer. Slurry concentration profiles can be derived from either in-situ [1] or non-intrusive [2] measurements. Although concentration data can be obtained throughout the mixer via either of these approaches, is not possible to differentiate between *individual* size fractions for a mixture of particle sizes. Most of the reported studies on slurry mixing involve measurements on monodisperse suspensions. In reality, however, it is more common to find a range of particle sizes in a plant-scale mixer. There is, therefore, a need to obtain data on the distribution of solids for a polydisperse suspension for design purposes. This provided the incentive for the investigation described in this chapter in which Positron Emission Tomography (PET) was used to follow the mixing of a slurry mixture containing two different particle sizes (i.e. bimodal).

PET produces images of high resolution (8 mm in the x, y and z-planes) but, in contrast to electrical-based tomography techniques, requires longer time for data acquisition and image reconstruction. The technique was exploited as part of this research programme to assess the *feasibility* of applying PET to obtain quantitative data on slurry mixing processes. Experiments were performed using the PET camera at the University of Birmingham, which is the only such facility in the world dedicated to process engineering applications. A detailed description of the methodology and applications of the technique can be found in the preceding chapter by Parker et al. [3].

All the measurements reported in this chapter were performed on a small-scale mixing tank of capacity 5 dm^3. Mono and bimodal sand-water slurries were agitated at different impeller speeds to examine the effect of impeller speed on the homogeneity of solids in the mixer. The study described in this chapter illustrates that PET *can* provide distribution data on particles within a specified size range. The research is significant because it represents the first attempt to visualize slurry mixing with this technique, in which small diameter particles are labelled.

2.0 Tomographic reconstruction of images

PET uses a positron-emitting radioisotope to act as a tracer within the opaque slurry mixture. The positrons annihilate with neighbouring electrons to generate high energy γ-ray photons. Each annihilation creates a single pair of 511 keV γ-rays, which travel in diametrically opposite directions. This pair of γ-rays are detected as coincident counts in two position-sensitive detectors and each coincident event is logged on computer. Coincident detection of these γ-rays on either side of the field of view suggests that the annihilation must have occurred on the line joining the two detection points. Detection of many lines then allows 3-D image reconstruction of the distribution of the labelled particulates within the slurry mixture, thus allowing quantification of particle concentration.

The Birmingham PET camera employs two detectors (600 x 300 mm^2) which can be separated by a distance of up to 600 mm. These detectors are gas-filled multi-wire proportional counter detectors [4]. In the experiments reported here, the detectors were separated by a distance of 300 mm. Normally, to fully sample the activity distribution, the detectors would have to be rotated but for these mixing experiments axial symmetry and steady-state conditions were assumed.

While travelling through matter, in this case the slurry mixture, a γ-ray may be subject to attenuation effects due to absorption or scattering. As discussed in the previous chapter, correction for attenuation is straightforward. The detected photon end points, along each line, form a vector through the 3-D space between the detectors. This vector is back-projected through a 3-D array. Each element in the array represents a small cube of space (a voxel). To build up an activity distribution, many vectors are back-projected. Prior to back-projection, weighting is applied to each coincident event to correct for attenuation along its line of sight. If insufficiently known, this attenuation can be measured using an external source in a technique developed by McNeil [5]. The back-projected image contains tails due to the reconstruction process. These tails can be removed using a deconvolution process. Details about the theoretical and practical aspects associated with the deconvolution and attenuation procedures have been described by McNeil [5].

3.0 Experimental details

In this study a flat-based mixing tank of standard geometry was seated on a platform within the detection area of the PET camera as shown in Fig.1. Sieve fractions of sand with diameters in the size range 150-210 μm and 600-710 μm were agitated separately at a mean concentration of 6.3% by volume (C_m). For mixing of bimodal slurry suspensions two compositions were considered. One contained 20% wt 150-210 μm and 80% wt 600-710 μm. The second contained 80% wt 150-210 μm and 20% wt 600-710 μm.

Agitation was provided by a 6-bladed Rushton turbine ($D = T/2$) with an impeller clearance of $T/4$ where D is the vessel diameter and T is the height of the slurry in the tank. All the measurements were performed under steady-state conditions and the data capture time was 30 minutes per impeller speed.

In all the experiments, a small fraction of the sand, typically 250 mg, was labelled with ^{18}F in a cyclotron. In the series of experiments using bimodal mixtures, the largest sieve fraction (600-710 μm) was labelled. Prior to introducing the tracer, the exact coordinates of the vessel boundary were established by positioning a point source of a ^{22}Na at locations around the circumference.

Images were reconstructed into a 64 x 64 x 64 array of 0.6 x 0.6 x 0.6 cm³ voxels, assuming axial symmetry about the central axis. The axis position was found separately for each run using the point source location data. Correction for attenuation was made by assuming the vessel to be equivalent to a uniform cylinder of water. Each image was then normalized to estimate the solids volume fraction within each voxel, using the following procedure: The content (number of counts) of a voxel xyz in the raw image w_{xyz} was converted into the volume fraction of solids within a voxel C_{xyz} using the relationship $\Sigma\, v_v\, C_{xyz} = V_T$ (where v_v is the volume of each voxel) and V_T is the total volume of sand. Therefore, $\Sigma\, C_{xyz} = V_T/v_v$ and each raw image was normalized by a factor $V_T/(v_v\, \Sigma\, w_{xyz})$. For the monosize dispersion, the volume for normalization was 0.063 x 4000 cm³ but with the bimodal runs the volume to which each image was normalized was (0.2 or 0.8) x 0.063 x 4000 cm³.

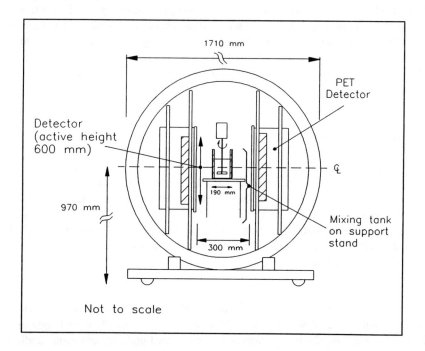

Fig.1 *Experimental arrangement for study of slurry mixing using PET*

4.0 Results

The image data provided by the back-projection algorithm were imported into the Tomographic Data Viewer (TDV) software package, Jia et al. [6]. This package was specifically designed to display and analyse tomography data in various formats, hence easing image interpretation. Fig 2 shows one typical screen mode (3-D mesh format) in the TDV incorporating slice images of the coarse (600-710 μm) slurry mixture at different impeller speeds. The array of images in Fig.3 was obtained using tomography data for the slurries with a bimodal composition. Two impeller speeds were employed for the coarse bimodal (20% 150-210 μm and 80% 600-710 μm) and the fine bimodal (80% 150-210 μm and 20% 600-710 μm) slurries.

The extent of homogeneity within a mixing vessel can be quantified in terms of a Mixing Index MI [1,2]. This index provides a measure of the deviation of solids concentration from the mean throughout the vessel. As the extent of homogeneity increases, the value tends to zero at perfect mixing. The mixing index for a single image plane can be defined as:

$$MI_{AT} = \frac{1}{C_m} \left(\frac{1}{(n_s - 1)} \sum_{t=1}^{n_s} (C_{xyz} - C_m)^2 \right)^{\frac{1}{2}} \qquad (1)$$

where:

MI_{AT} =   Mixing Index for axial concentration profile obtained from tomography measurements

C_{xyz} =   the solids concentration in voxel xyz

C_m =   the mean solids concentration

n_s =   the number of measurement sample positions.

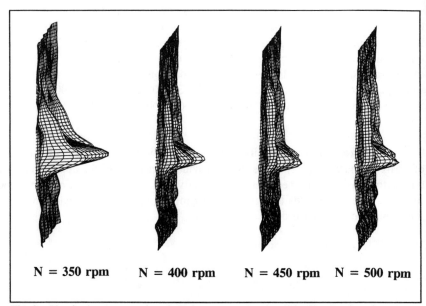

Fig.2 Vertical cross-section 3-D image mesh of solids distribution for coarse slurry mixture at different impeller speeds.

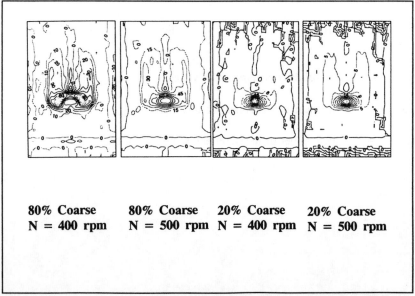

Fig.3 2-D contour of solids distribution for bimodal slurry mixtures at different impeller speeds. Values of volume fraction (x1000) shown on contours.

4.1 Agitation of coarse slurry mixture

The coarse slurry mixture comprised particles in the size range 600-710 μm. Four agitation rates were considered. The initial activity of the labelled sand was 475 μC.

The minimum agitator speed required for complete suspension of a slurry is often referred to as the "just suspension speed" (N_{JS}) and indicates the speed at which no particle remains stationary on the base for more than 1-2 s [7]. The N_{JS} value of the coarse slurry was estimated from the Zweitering correlation [7] to be 505 rpm. Fig.2 shows the solids volume fraction distribution throughout the mixer for impeller speeds of 350, 400, 450 and 500 rpm. All these speeds are below N_{JS} and, as expected, each image shows that the solids were inadequately suspended resulting in a highly non-uniform vertical distribution of particles. Therefore, a large portion of the sand remains in the region of the impeller. This non-uniformity is most apparent at the low impeller speed of 350 rpm.

Axial concentration profiles at each of the impeller speeds are plotted in Fig.4. These profiles were obtained using quantitative image data at a radial position of 7 voxels off-centre from the impeller axis (i.e. at 42 mm from the axis).

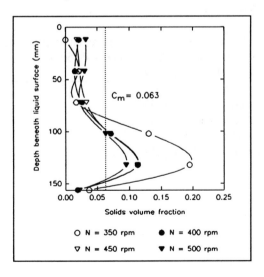

Fig.4 *Axial concentration profiles for 600-710 μm sand measured using PET.*

Quantitative interpretation of these profiles is evident by plotting the data as impeller speed versus homogeneity index MI_{AT} (Fig.5). MI_{AT} represents the mixing index for the axial profile calculated using tomography data. It is clear from this figure that as the mixing speed increases the extent of homogeneity is also increased. The only contrast in terms of MI_{AT} is achieved between the impeller speeds of 350 rpm and 400 rpm. This is verified in the tomographic images (Fig.2). Between the impeller speeds of 400 and 500 rpm there is little variation in MI, which is also verified in the corresponding images.

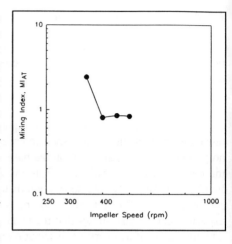

Fig.5   *Variation of MI_{AT} with impeller speed for 600-710 μm sand.*

4.2 Agitation of fine slurry mixture

As with the coarse slurry mixtures, four agitation rates were used to suspend the 150-210 μm sand-water slurry: 300, 350, 400 and 450 rpm. The labelled sand had an initial activity of 490 μC. The N_{JS} value, determined from the Zweitering correlation [7], was 390 rpm. According to the original 2-D slice images [2] all the sand appeared well distributed throughout the slurry volume for each impeller speed.

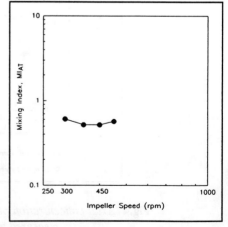

This is borne out in Fig.6. There is little variation in the MI_{AT} with speed (0.61 at 300 rpm and 0.57 at 450 rpm). This suggests that the $T/2$ impeller provides a good distribution for such a small sand size.

Fig. 6 *MI_{AT} vs impeller speed for 150-210 μm sand.*

4.3 Agitation of bimodal slurry mixtures

In examining the suspension of the bimodal mixtures, it should be remembered that the coarse fraction of sand was always labelled for each experimental run. Fig.3 shows the distribution of *coarse* sand in the mixing vessel for each of the bimodal mixtures at each of the impeller speeds (400 and 500 rpm). It is evident from the images of the coarse bimodal slurry (80% 600-710 μm fraction and 20% 150-210 μm) that there is an axial variation in solids distribution with solids concentrated in the impeller region. Fig.7 illustrates this quantitatively. For both impeller speeds of 400 and 500 rpm the particulate solids are more concentrated in the impeller region. With the bimodal mixture composed of 20% 600-710 μm fraction and 80% 150-210 μm the trends are similar (Fig.7). The concentration profiles for this mixture (figure 7) show that of the fraction of coarse particles, the peak occurs in the impeller region.

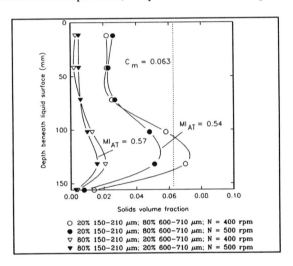

Fig.7 *Axial concentration profile of individual sieve fraction*
(600-710 μm) in a bimodal slurry mixture.

Fig.7 also shows the MI_{AT} values for two of the distribution profiles of coarse sand. In computing these MI_{AT} values the mean volume fraction of the 600-710 μm sand in the bimodal mixture was used.

5.0 Conclusions

This work represents the first reported use of PET for visualizing slurry mixing. The results are congruent with those obtained from independent measurements using alternative tomographic methods such as electrical resistance tomography [8]. The distribution of solids is more homogeneous as impeller speed is increased. Results from the bimodal slurry mixture confirm that the spatial distribution of an individual sieve fraction can be obtained satisfactorily. For the same impeller speed, the degree of homogeneity is higher for slurries containing more fines than coarse particles, as one might expect.

The potential significance of the PET method has been demonstrated and it is apparent that PET data could assist in development of advanced theoretical and practical models of mixing processes. For instance, the homogeneity index for an individual sieve fraction can be computed. Ideally, knowledge of the variation of this index with a *range* of volume fractions and particle sizes at different impeller speeds would be most beneficial for design purposes. There is a great need to determine the distribution of an individual sieve fraction in a mixture of sizes. Data of this nature would be particularly valuable in minerals processing. The information could be used, for example, to predict the effect of different densities and sizes on segregation in gravity separation-based processes. One such example is hydraulic classification which involves separation of particles, of different size and density, by virtue of settling velocities. Particles are passed into an elutriator which has an upward flow of fluid. The lightest particles rise with the fluid while the heaviest fall. The ability to map the distribution of mineral solids of different densities and sizes would be a useful aid to this equipment design. It is hoped to develop these concepts in future work.

Notation

C_m Mean volume fraction of solids
C_{xyz} Volume fraction of solids in voxel (x,y,z)
D Impeller diameter (m)
MI Mixing Index
MI_{AT} Mixing Index for axial concentration profile obtained from tomography measurements
N_{JS} Just suspension speed (rev s^{-1})
v_v Volume of voxel (m^3)
V_T Total volume of sand (m^3)
w_{xyz} Number of counts in voxel xyz (C)

References

[1]   A.T.C. Mak, PhD Thesis, University College London (1992).
[2]   S.L. McKee, PhD Thesis, UMIST (1994).

[3]   D.J. Parker, D.M. Benton, P. Fowles, P.A. McNeil and Min Tan (1995) (in this volume).

[4]   M.R. Hawkesworth, M.A. O'Dwyer, J. Walker, P. Fowles, J. Heritage, P.A.E. Stewart, R.C. Witcomb, J.E. Bateman, J.F. Connolly, and R. Stephenson, Nucl. Instr. and Meth. A253 (1986) p 145.

[5]   P.A. McNeil, PhD Thesis, University of Birmingham (1994).

[6]   X. Jia, R.A. Williams, F.J. Dickin and S.L. McKee, Process Tomography - 1995 - Implementation for Industrial Processes, ed. M.S. Beck et al. (UMIST, Manchester, 1995) p 371.

[7]   Th.N. Zweitering, Chem.Eng.Sci., 8 (1958) p 244.

[8]   R.A. Williams, X. Jia and S.L. McKee, Powder Technol. (1995) in press.

Chapter 22

Monitoring Cyclone Performance using Resistance Tomography

R A Williams
Particle & Colloid Engineering Group
Camborne School of Mines
University of Exeter
Redruth, Cornwall TR15 3SE U.K.

F J Dickin, A Guiterrez and M S Beck
Department of Electrical Engineering & Electronics
University of Manchester Institute of Science & Technology
PO Box 88, Manchester M60 1QD U.K.

M. Wang, O.M. Ilyas and T. Dyakowksi
Department of Chemical Engineering
University of Manchester Institute of Science & Technology
PO Box 88, Manchester M60 1QD U.K.

1. Introduction

The *operation* and *control* of hydrocyclones and dense medium cyclones for particle sizing, density-based separations and dewatering duties has received little attention, despite the widespread use of such separators in the processing of chemicals, foodstuffs and mineral products. A number of problems can be encountered during routine operation, for example:

(i)   Gross malfunction can occur if the underflow orifice (apex), or occasionally the overflow exit, becomes blocked due to the presence of over-size particles or debris (such as wood chippings or wire).

(ii)   Variations in the feed materials (solid concentration, particle size distribution, mineralogical composition, volumetric flow rate) may modify the separation characteristics. A few proprietary cyclones are reconfigurable for control purposes, by allowing the diameter of the overflow (or vortex finder insert) or the apex diameter to be adjusted (via an concentric inflatable rubber ring valve). Other methods include the admission of wash-water in the apex region and the back-pressuring of the overflow exit. A method of monitoring the changes in the feed properties or its consequences on separator performance is needed in order to actuate any control operation. Whilst changes to the feed rate can be achieved by using a variable speed pump or closing down one or more feed lines to a bank of cyclones, this is not widely practised. Water additions can be made more easily, although this may not be desirable, e.g. in dewatering applications.

(iii)   Separator performance can drift with time, or suddenly, as the internal surfaces of the cyclone become worn due to the abrasive action of solids, or thermal or chemically-enhanced degradation of the wall materials. The vortex finder and apex are particularly vulnerable to wear. The progressive loss of process efficiency can be subtle, sometimes extending over several weeks of operation thus impairing detection on a shift-by-shift basis by process operators. Progressive deterioration in classification performance can cause problems, for example, in banks of hydrocyclones that are used to prepare 'backfill' slurry prior to pumping down to underground cavities for long-term storage.

(iv)   The transition from a *spray* to a *rope* underflow discharge is often accompanied by a marked change is classification performance. The nature of the efflux of slurry from the underflow of a hydrocyclone depends on the properties of the feed slurry and the separator performance. For instance, for size classification duties, hydrocyclones treating dense slurries are best operated close to the roping condition but not actually roping. In the roping state the axial air core present in the cyclone disappears, the cut size increases markedly and the pressure drop across the cyclone is reduced.

Various methods have been proposed to provide on- and off-line detection of the above malfunctions, as reviewed elsewhere [1]. The measurement challenge is compounded by the fact that many plants processing ultrafine industrial minerals and metal ores might employ banks of cyclones of various diameters, each containing from five up to several hundred units. The present contribution will be confined to reviewing previous applications of tomographic methods for measuring the behaviour of different types of stationary-body centrifugal separators. Recent developments in the use of one method, based on electrical resistance sensors, is considered in detail for on-line monitoring of hydrocyclone and dense medium separators.

2. Status of Applications of Tomography to Cyclone Separators

Of the few applications of tomographic technology, most have been directed towards providing data for the purposes of verifying theoretical and empirical model predictions of fluid flow and the distribution of solids within regions inside separators. Previously such measurements could only be obtained at discrete points in the separator, requiring great experimental ingenuity, using conventional invasive mechanical, electrical or optical sensors [2].

One of the first convincing feasibility demonstrations of the application of a tomographic method utilized X-ray computed tomography (XCT) to examine the two dimensional images of the coal and shale *off-line* in a sample taken from the float and sink product streams from a dense medium separator, from which the coal washability could be computed [3]. Subsequently, *on-line* time-averaged images of the solid concentration profiles and location of slurry, froth and air interfaces in a cross-section through an air-sparged hydrocyclone flotation were obtained [4], as reported in detail elsewhere in this volume. Solid concentration profiles obtained using X-ray photography (rather than tomography) have been reported [5] and compared with predictions from fluid flow models. The use of hard field sensors (see Chapter 4) has considerable attractions in providing a high resolution image, but is less practical, at the present time, for routine use in an industrial environment. Further, the temporal resolution may often be inadequate to probe fluctuations in the flow structure inside the cyclone.

The development of electrical resistance tomography (ERT) for use on industrial processes also allows the interior of the cyclone to be probed but employing a more rapid imaging speed but with a consequent trade-off in spatial resolution. The principles of ERT instruments and their performance has been described in detail previously [6,7] including the feasibility of incorporating sensors into metal-walled process vessels [8]. These methods are reaching a sufficient level of maturity to begin to enable measurement of steady-state slurry concentration profiles in stirred tanks and cyclones for comparison with advanced computational fluid dynamic predictions [9-11]. The wealth of data delivered by ERT promises to allow the generation of three-dimensional maps by using multi-planes of sensors which may result in a radically different approach to modelling and intelligent on-line control of processes.

Electrical sensing methods based on dielectric contrast using electrical capacitance tomography (ECT) have been used on cyclones to analyse oil-water separators [12], in which the continuous phase is essentially electrically non-conducting (oil). ECT has also be used to measure the nature of the discharge from hydrocyclone underflow using external sensors mounted beneath the hydrocyclone [13]. The principle of using the image data from two planes of capacitance sensors to measure the diameter, angle of discharge and time-varying fluctuations of the former for on-line monitoring and control of cyclone operation was suggested. Such a method could be used to detect several of the fault conditions (i-iv, listed in Section 1) based on interpretative models incorporating process parameters (slurry properties, production rates, historical data) derived from statistical analysis (principal components analysis and multivariate methods).

3. On-line Monitoring of Cyclone Behaviour

Two illustrations of the use of ERT for monitoring the behaviour of two types of separator are described below. The measurements were performed on a 44 mm (internal) diameter hydrocyclone (Mozley, Redruth) and a laboratory-scale *large diameter coal dense medium separator* (LARCODEMS).

3.1 Air-core size and movement in a dense medium cyclone separator

The laboratory-scale LARCODEMS unit (150 mm diameter, 450 mm length) was fitted with two planes of sixteen ERT sensors (Fig. 1). Measurements were made with a UMIST Mk.1b ERT system using an adjacent electrode current injection protocol [6,7]. Data were reconstructed using, for the results presented here, a 'qualitative' reconstruction algorithm [7] based on a finite element method using a circular-shaped mesh with 564 triangular elements to allow definition of the gas-slurry boundaries [14]. Equation (1) is a representation of the sensitivity density coefficient algorithm; $P(k)$ denotes the grey-scale value of pixel k centred at co-ordinates (x,y) with reference to the relative change of conductivity at that pixel.

$$P(k) = \frac{\Delta\sigma'_k}{\sigma} = \frac{\displaystyle\sum_{i=1}^{N-1}\sum_{j=i+1}^{N} D_{i,j,k}\ln\left[\frac{V'_{i,j}}{V_{i,j}}\right]}{\displaystyle\sum_{i=1}^{N-1}\sum_{j=i+1}^{N} D_{i,j,k}} \tag{1}$$

$V'(i,j)$ is the voltage measurement from electrode j after a conductivity change occurred inside the separator when injecting current at electrode i whereas $V(i,j)$ is the measurement prior to any change. N is the number of electrodes employed in the strategy - in this case sixteen. $D_{i,j,k}$ denotes the sensitivity density at pixel k which is defined as $D_{i,j,k} = \nabla\phi_{i,k}\cdot\nabla\varphi_{j,k}$ in which $\phi_{i,k}$ and $\phi_{j,k}$ are the potentials at pixel k with respect to the currents injected at electrodes i and j respectively.

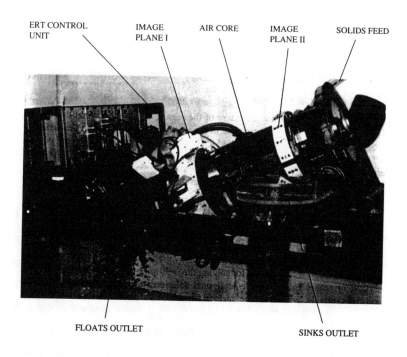

ERT CONTROL
UNIT

IMAGE
PLANE I

AIR CORE

IMAGE
PLANE II

SOLIDS FEED

FLOATS OUTLET

SINKS OUTLET

(a)

Medium inlet

Raw feed

Clean coal

Reject

(b)

Fig. 1: (a) Photograph of instrumented laboratory scale LARCODEMS unit and (b) schematic diagram showing principal feed and products streams in coal-shale separation

Unlike X-rays, which follow a pencil-beam trajectory through the subject, electric current traverses a non-linear path of least resistance. As a consequence, the distribution of pixel sensitivities throughout the region of interest is non-uniform. A compensation method based on Gaussian profiling was employed to limit this effect in which the maximum value of pixel intensity, P_{max}, is multiplied by an empirically derived weighting parameter b [14]:

$$\overline{P}_{max} = P_{max} \cdot e^{-b\hat{r}^2} \tag{2}$$

where $\hat{r}$ is the radial position normalised for a circular domain of unit radius. A relation was found between the diameter of the air-core and the pixel intensities:

$$d_1 \approx d_0 \cdot \left(\frac{\overline{P}_{max,1}}{\overline{P}_{max,0}}\right)^{\mu} \quad \overline{P}_{max} = P_{max} \cdot e^{-b\hat{r}^2} \tag{3}$$

where d_0, $\overline{P}_{max,0}$ are the diameter and image intensity of a reference 'air-core' from a non-conductive rod and d_1, $\overline{P}_{max,1}$ are those for the real air-core. The value of the constant μ was found to be around 0.5-0.6. In the case of an air-core located exactly at the axis of the separator, the intensity of its image can be regarded as being that of a Gaussian profile. The region of related intensity changes in the central region of the image, as a result of back-projection, is larger than the actual size of the air-core but maintains its original shape (Fig. 2). The shaded area at the cut-point denoted by position B'-C' in Fig. 2 is similar to that of the actual air-core shown in the B-C plane. An estimation method based on comparison with the actual size of the air-core was adopted to find this cut-point or 'filtering point' for scaling the air-core inside centrifugal separators. However, the estimation method cannot be used in practice for accurate scaling ($<$ 5% error) due to the changes of the process and measurement environment, such as the current amplitude used and the electrolyte conductivity of the slurry under investigation. The optimum algorithm was based on a comparison between the boundary voltage profile acquired from the test vessel and that simulated using the finite element method model with the conductivity distribution at the sequentially renewed cut-cross-section, so as to approach a minimum difference between the two profiles. In order to prevent the divergent solution and reduce the error within the algorithm from measurement singularity, the difference between two relative profile changes was employed in the algorithm.

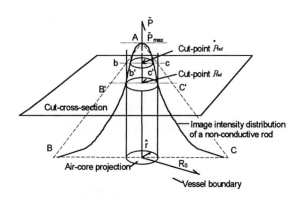

Fig. 2: Determination of the cut cross-section in the air-core scaling method

In practice, the image intensity distribution is first approximated to a triangle ABC as shown in Fig. 2. Then an initial cut-point is selected at a cut-point P_{cut}^{*} (shown by the line b-c) determined using the simple triangular relationship:

$$P_{cut}^{*} = \overline{P}_{max} \cdot (1 - \hat{r}) \qquad (4)$$

where $\hat{r}$ is the normalised radius given by $d/(2R_{0})$, d is the unknown diameter of the air-core which is obtained from equation (3). The projection area obtained by the cut-point is smaller than the real value ($\overline{b'c'} < \overline{bc}$), or the cut-point P_{cut}^{*} is larger than the correct one P_{cut}. A search factor, k, was employed to help to reduce the cut-point gradually:

$$\overline{P}_{cut}^{*} = k \cdot \overline{P}_{max} \cdot (1 - \hat{r}) \qquad (k < 1) \qquad (5)$$

A series of conductivity distributions at different cross-sections were obtained when the search factor was gradually reduced. The boundary voltages, U', were simulated by substituting a conductivity distribution into the FEM forward solution

14]. Comparing a series of relative changes of boundary voltages between those from imulation and measurements, V', as given in equation (6), an optimum projection area or the air-core image was obtained.

$$\vartheta = \sum_{i=1}^{N-1} \sum_{j=i+1}^{N} \left[\frac{V'_{i,j}}{V_{i,j}} - \frac{U'_{i,j}}{U_{i,j}} \right]^2 \qquad (6)$$

where V, U are boundary voltages respectively for measurement and simulation in a homogeneous conductivity distribution.

A series of images depicting the collapse of a stable air core (induced by a decrease in the volumetric feed flow rate) in the laboratory-scale LARCODEM at the sensing plane I closest to the floats product (Fig 1) is shown in Fig. 3. The size, shape and position of the air-core undergoes violent oscillation and eventually breaks ups. ERT can be used to capture these fast processes.

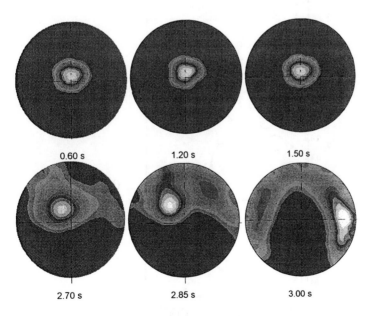

| 0.60 s | 1.20 s | 1.50 s |
| 2.70 s | 2.85 s | 3.00 s |

Fig. 3: Dynamics of air-core collapse induced by a sudden reduction in feed flow to LARCODEMS. Lighter regions correspond to higher resistivity (gas phase). Images obtained at sensing plane I (Fig. 2).

Fig. 4 also depicts, in a graphical form, the dynamics of air-core collapse in a separate experiment as the feed flow rate (Q) is reduced over a 2 s period. Here the data abstracted from the images have been presented in the form of the dimensionless air core diameter σ_0 (given by dividing the imaged air core spherical equivalent diameter by the cyclone body diameter). The dimensionless eccentricity ε is also plotted (given by dividing the distance of the centre of the gravity of the air core to the geometric centre of the cyclone by the cyclone body radius.) The air-core at electrode plane II disappeared after 1.6 s (after which point the electrodes were in contact with air owing to the very low liquid level) and after 1.2 s for electrode plane I (when the air-core was replaced by liquid). Note that the eccentricity of the air core (Fig. 4c, plane II) suggests an increasing instability as the flow rate (Fig.4a) is reduced below a critical value. It may be postulated that the eccentricity could be used as a means of monitoring air-core instability and that values above $\varepsilon = 0.1$ should be avoided [2].

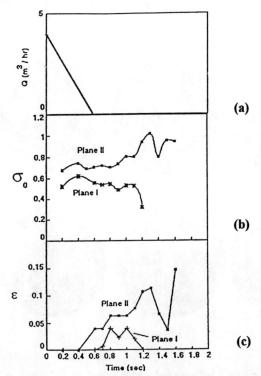

Fig. 4: Interpretation of ERT images showing dynamics of air-core collapse in a laboratory LARCODEMS as feed flow is reduced suddenly (a) showing corresponding dimensionless air core diameter (b) and eccentricity (c)

3.2 Underflow discharge control in a hydrocyclone

Measurements of air core dynamics and resistivity images which can be used to infer the solid concentration in a plane through a hydrocyclone can be acquired in a similar way to those described above. Fig. 5 shows a sequence of images (each snapshot corresponding to 50 ms of data acquisition time) obtained with a UMIST Mk2a DSP-based ERT system, at a cross-section just below the feed inlet of the 44 mm diameter hydrocyclone. Reconstructed data for different feed rates and feed concentrations from water up to 35 % calcium silicate by weight. As the slurry concentration is increased an annular region of solids (shown by the darker region) is observed to form. Note also that the air core (the central white regions) is often irregular in shape and eccentric.

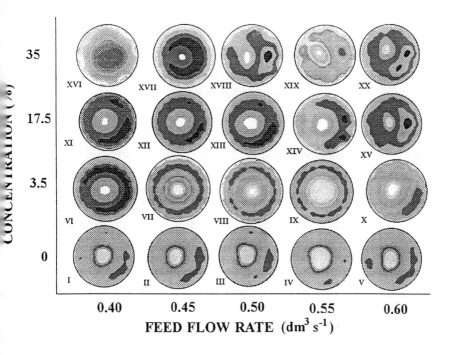

Fig. 5: Sequence of resistivity images of hydrocyclone cross section just below feed inlet for different feed flow rates and solid concentrations (by % wt)

Such data is useful for verifying CFD simulations and predictions of the air core size. For instance, by analysing the image sets (as described in 3.1) the air core size can be elucidated. Fig. 6 shows such a plot of the percentage of the cross-sectional area occupied by the air core *vs.* flow rate. The air core increases with volumetric throughput and decreases as the slurry density is increased.

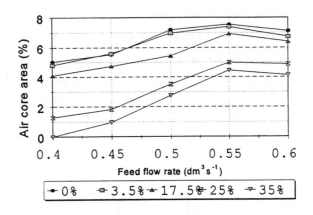

Fig. 6: Apparent area occupied by air core as a function of feed flow rate and concentration of solids.

The air core size reflects the nature of discharge from the hydrocyclone (see section 1). Hence the information in the ERT image can be correlated with separator performance, as shown in Fig. 7. The two states of roping and spray discharge also exhibit different temporal stability (causing different fluctuations in air core to be observed) and the nature of the rotational movement of the discharge is related to slurry viscosity etc. ERT images can be interpreted to allow fault recognition (as in Fig 7) - the characteristics of the air core size, eccentricity and time fluctuations are distinctive, allowing roping to be recognised.

Work on more quantitative analysis is in progress, where the ERT signatures are to be correlated against process performance (cut size, solid content, separator efficiency, throughput, discharge angle etc.).

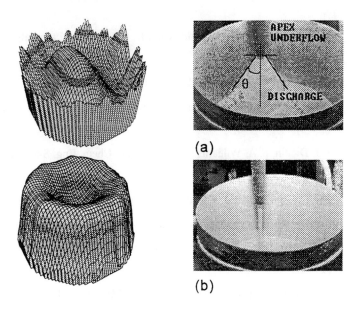

Fig. 7: Isometric view of resistivity tomograms (left hand column) and photographs of underflow discharge (right hand column) for (a) 3.5 wt % and (b) 35 wt % slurries in 44 mm diameter hydrocyclone for feed rate of 0.5 dm³ s⁻¹ .

4. Future Prospects

The use of ERT for multiphase flow imaging offers considerable potential for flow modelling, separator design and on-line process monitoring. This contribution has sought to demonstrate the particular case of condition monitoring for cyclonic separators which provides one example of a number of possible applications in separation technology.

5. References

[1]   R.A. Williams, P.J. Gregory, D. Brown, P. James and N. Parkinson, submitted for publication (1995).

[2]   R.A. Williams, O.M. Ilyas and T. Dyakowski, Coal Preparation **15** 149-163 (1995).

[3]   C. Lin, J.D. Miller, A.B. Cortes and R. Galery, Coal Preparation, 9 107-119
       (1992).

[4]   C. Lin, J.D. Miller and A. Cortes, KONA, 10 88-95 (1992).

[5]   K.P. Galvin and J.B. Smitham, Minerals Engineering, 7 (10) 1269-1280
       (1995).

[6]   F.J. Dickin, R.A. Williams and M.S. Beck, Chem. Eng. Sci., 48 1883-1897
       (1993).

[7]   R.A. Williams and M.S. Beck (eds.) Process Tomography - Principles,
       Techniques and Applications, (Butterworth-Heinemann, Oxford, 1995).

[8]   M.Wang, F.J. Dickin and R.A. Williams, Electronic Letters, 30 771-773
       (1994).

[9]   S.L. McKee, Ph.D. Thesis, University of Manchester Institute of Science &
       Technology, 1994.

[10]   T. Dyakowski and R.A. Williams, Powder Technol. (1995) in press.

[11]   R.A. Williams, X. Jia and S.L. McKee, Powder Technol. (1995) in press.

[12]   E.A. Hammer, Private Communication (1995), displayed at European
       Concerted Action Meeting on Process Tomography, Bergen, Norway, April
       1995.

[13]   R.A. Williams, T. Dyakowski, C.G. Xie, S.P. Luke, P.J. Gregory, R.B.
       Edwards and L.F. Gate, in Process Tomography - Implementation for
       Industrial Processes, ed. M.S. Beck et al., (EU/UMIST, Manchester, 1995)
       p3-15.

[14]   M. Wang, Ph.D. Thesis, University of Manchester Institute of Science &
       Technology, 1994.

Chapter 23

Analysis of Liquid Flow Distribution in a Trickle Bed Reactor

D. Toye, P. Marchot, M.Crine, G. L'Homme
Laboratoire de génie chimique, Institut de Chimie - B6
University of Liège, B-4000 Liège, Belgium

1. Introduction

The hydrodynamics of the gas-liquid flow in trickle-bed reactors is very intricate. Up to now, rather few models are able to cope with the complexity of the mechanisms which govern this phenomenon. Some attempts in this direction have been reported in the literature [1, 2]. None of these attempts is able to give a complete description of :

- the local hydrodynamic phenomena in terms of local packing properties,
- the spatial fluctuations of these phenomena due to the packing heterogeneity,
- the relation between the local phenomena and what we may observe at the level of the whole packing.

There is obviously a lack of experimental information which would give us a better insight into these complex mechanisms. The objective of this paper is to present the feasibility of a new technique based on x-ray transmission through a trickle flow column. It consists of x-ray tomography applied to the determination of the spatial distribution of the gas-liquid-solid phase saturation in a cross section of the column. This technique is applied to a trickling filter, which is one of the main biological reactor used for the secondary treatment of waste waters.

2. Description of the Technique

X-ray tomography refers to the cross-sectional imaging of an object from data collected by irradiating this object with x-ray coplanar beams from many different directions. The x-ray intensity attenuation is directly proportional to the density of the medium through which the radiation is transmitted, i.e., to the different phase hold-ups. The measure of a transmitted beam intensity yields a linear averaged value of the attenuation coefficients along a given ray. Local values of these attenuation coefficients may be estimated by tomographic numerical techniques.

This technique of measurement presents several advantages : it is a true *in-situ* non-invasive technique, its spatial resolution is very good (between 1 and 2 mm), and it provides information about the local packing morphology and the local structure of the liquid flow.

Among the large number of mathematical approaches that have been used for image reconstruction [3], we have chosen the two-dimensional Fourier method, which is an analytic method based on exact mathematical solutions of the image equations. The theoretical basis of this reconstruction algorithm is the Fourier Slice Theorem according to which the one-dimensional Fourier transform of a parallel projection is equal to a slice of the two-dimensional Fourier transform of the original object [4]. The reconstruction algorithm accounts for the particular geometry of our scanning set-up (fan beam geometry).

3. Experimental Scanning Setup

The x-ray tomographic set-up had to satisfy two main constraints: It had to be rotated around a vertical axis in order to provide scans of horizontal cross sections of the packing, and it had to be able to record x-ray transmission through rather large trickle flow columns.

The experimental set-up installed in our laboratory allows scanning of columns whose maximum size is 0.8 m in diameter and 2 m in height. The x-ray scanner has been built from different constitutive elements available on the market.

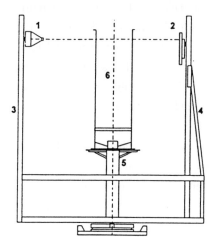

Fig. 1 Experimental set-up

The main parts of this set-up are represented in Figure 1. The x-ray source (1) is a point source generator, producing a 40° fan beam of x-rays, whose energy can be varied from 0 to 160 kV (Balteau-Schlumberger, Belgium). The detector (2) is constituted by a linear array of 1024 photodiodes (Balteau-Schlumberger, Belgium). The x-ray source and the detector are supported by two pillars ((3) and (4)) of a metallic structure. Their vertical displacement along these 2 pillars is perfectly synchronized.

The metallic structure rotates around a plate (5) supporting the packed column (6) and the fluid feed and discharge devices. During a rotation of 360°, a large number (>1024) of projections are recorded. At the end of a rotation, more than one million intensity values are available. The reconstructed images have a maximal size of 1024x1024 pixels.

The projection data are stored on a microcomputer and then sent to a second one (a PC equipped with a I860 card), on which the reconstruction algorithm is implemented. The computation time required by the reconstruction equals approximately 4 hours for 1024x1024 pixels images. In order to reduce the reconstruction time during the development phase, we have decided to limit our investigations to 512x512 pixel images.

The liquid is fed at the top of the packed column (6), whose dimensions are 0.6 m inner diameter and 2 m height. The column wall is made of polyethylene, characterized by a very low attenuation coefficient. The fixed bed is constituted by Etapak210 (Mass Transfer, UK), which is a random polypropylene packing. The main geometrical characteristics of this packing are a nominal diameter of approximately 0.05 m, a void fraction of 95% and a specific area equal to 220 m^2/m^3.

The liquid used is pure water, characterized by an attenuation coefficient 1000 larger than air. The water flow rate can be varied from 0 to 1000 l/h, corresponding to superficial velocities ranging from 0 to 10^{-3} m/s.

4.   Experimental Results

4.1. *Analysis of the packing morphology*

One of the first objectives of this study was to determine the packing morphological characteristics which control the liquid flow distribution. To this aim, we have first scanned the packed column without any liquid flow. The column wall thickness is about 0.015 m and despite the polyethylene low absorbance coefficient, its absorbance is high enough to cause halo effects close to the wall in the reconstructed images. In order to avoid this artifact, it is necessary to subtract, before the reconstruction, the projection signals obtained with an empty column from those obtained with the packed column. This subtraction is justified because of the linearity of x-ray attenuation.

Figure 2 represents an example of reconstructed section. This figure clearly evidences the non-uniformity of the distribution of the packing elements characterized by the presence of white zones in the section.

The physical soundness of the reconstructed images has been further evaluated by determining the overall void fraction and comparing it to the value announced by the manufacturer.

The void fractions have been calculated from images that had been normalized in such a way that the maximum pixel value equals 100%. The solid fractions resulting from these calculations are equal to about 5%, corresponding to a void fraction of 95%, i.e., exactly the value claimed by the manufacturer.

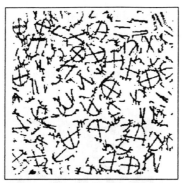

Fig. 2 Reconstructed image of a cross section of the packed column without liquid. Packing used: Etapak210 (Mass Transfer); Nominal diameter: 0.05 m; Threshold value: 20% of maximum pixel intensity.

The complexity of the packing morphology results mainly from the superposition of several characteristic scales [5]. This makes it rather difficult to understand the influence that this morphology exerts on the liquid hydrodynamics.

In this paper, we will focus our attention on the properties which characterize the random distribution of the packing elements within the column. In order to eliminate all the phenomena occurring at scales smaller than a given characteristic length we have to compute local averages. The size of the elementary cells over which these local averages have to be calculated may be determined by the correlation length of the spatial distribution of the individual pixel intensities. This correlation length is given by the first zero of the image autocorrelation function. It characterizes the details of the individual packing elements morphology. The correlation lengths obtained for the reconstructed sections of the packed column are about 7 pixels, i.e., 0.012 m.

Figure 3 shows the image obtained by locally averaging Fig. 2 over 7x7 pixel squares. It thus represents the spatial distribution of the locally averaged solid fractions. The geometrical details of the packing elements have been removed, but heterogeneities at the bed scale remain (white zones). These heterogeneities are essential characteristics of the packing texture which may affect the liquid flow distribution.

The spatial distribution of locally averaged solid fractions may be represented by a histogram, as illustrated on Fig. 4b. In the absence of any spatial correlation at the bed scale, this histogram should exhibit an exponential shape [6]. That is indeed the trend observed for the highest classes. The main difference concerns the two first classes. The jump observed between these two classes is thus an important feature of the distribution which translates the existence of spatial correlation at the bed scale.

Fig. 3 Reconstructed image of a cross section of the packed column without liquid, locally averaged over 7x7 pixel squares.

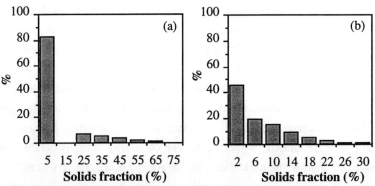

Fig. 4 Distribution of solid fraction: (a) without any local averaging, (b) locally averaged over 7x7 pixel squares.

One may note that averaging the pixel intensities over larger and larger areas would result in an elimination of any spatial correlation. But, in this case, both the experimental and theoretical histograms would be progressively transformed into a gaussian, due to the central limit theorem [7]. Fig. 4a shows the histogram obtained without any local averaging (individual pixel distribution). The discrepancies with respect to an exponential decrease are much more important because of an additional correlation at scales smaller or equal to the characteristic length of the packing elements. Actually in this case several distributions, occurring at different scales, are overlapping. This makes the phenomena much more difficult to analyze.

4.2. *Distribution of the liquid phase saturation*

The second objective of this study was to assess the feasibility of x-ray tomography to analyze the distribution of the gas and liquid phase saturations within the packed bed. To this aim, the trickling filter was fed with liquid by means of a multi-point source distributor. The scans have been realized in cross sections far enough from the top of the packing to avoid any inlet effect due to the distributor design.

After the image reconstruction, one may still observe artefacts resulting from the column wall column as already noticed with the dry packing. Furthermore, the attenuation coefficients of the liquid and solid phases are of the same order of magnitude. This makes it rather difficult to distinguish between the relative contributions of the two phases on the reconstructed images. In order to eliminate wall and packing contributions, the projection signals obtained with the drained packed bed have been subtracted from those recorded at the same column height with the irrigated packed bed. In such a way, the pixel intensities represent the sole contribution of the local liquid phase saturations.

In order to provide images of the distribution of the actual liquid phase saturations, it is necessary to convert pixel intensities into liquid saturations, i.e., to calibrate the scanning equipment. To this aim, mean values of the pixel intensities, calculated over the whole cross section, have been compared to macroscopic values of the liquid phase saturation determined on the same column (same diameter, same type of packing) by a tracer technique [8, 9]. The proportionality factor between the two quantities yields the calibration factor of the scanning equipment. Figure 5 represents an example of a calibrated image. This figure proves the non-uniformity of the distribution of the liquid phase. Preferential flow paths appear clearly on this picture. One should however note that a part only of the liquid films are actually represented on this figure. This is due to an automatic thresholding of the graphical representation: the absorbance of the thinnest films (a few tenths of millimeter) is lumped in the first grey level class with the noise signal. This could certainly be avoided by increasing the attenuation coefficient of the liquid phase, e.g., by adding lead or barium salts. Work is currently underway in that direction in our laboratory.

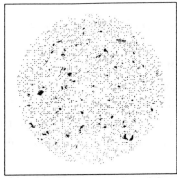

Fig. 5 Reconstructed image of a cross section of the column irrigated at a liquid flow rate of 6.10^{-4} m/s.

The estimates of the averaged liquid phase saturations determined by x-ray tomography have been compared with a partial wetting model [8]. The agreement is quite satisfactory. This model assumes a laminar flow over a part f_w of the packing. The wetting efficiency, f_w, is given by [8] :

$$f_w = \frac{Q}{Q + Q_{min}}$$

(Eq. 1)

where Q represents the liquid superficial velocity (in m/s). The minimum liquid superficial velocity, Q_{min}, is a measure of the packing wettability: the smaller Q_{min}, the better the solid wettability. For a laminar flow, it turns out that

$$h = k \cdot \frac{Q}{(Q + Q_{min})^{2/3}}$$

(Eq. 2)

where h represents the liquid phase saturation and k is a proportionality factor depending on the liquid and packing properties.

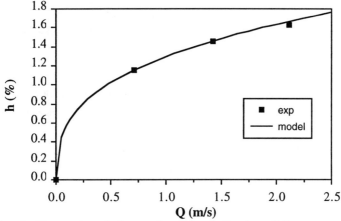

Fig. 6   Comparison between the x-ray estimates of the averaged liquid phase saturation and the prediction of a partial wetting model (Eq. 2).

The estimates of the parameters k and Qmin are 1.3×10^{-2} ($s^{1/3}$ $m^{-1/3}$) and 2.8×10^{-5} (m/s), respectively. These estimates may be compared with those obtained with a tracer technique, 1.3×10^{-2} ($s^{1/3}$ $m^{-1/3}$) and 1.1×10^{-4} (m/s), respectively. The difference between the two estimates of Q_{min} are probably due to different packing wettabilities.

5.   Conclusions

The results presented in this paper show that x-ray tomography is a very promising tool to investigate the complex hydrodynamic phenomena occurring within a trickling filter. It allows the experimental determination of the spatial distributions of the gas, liquid and solid phase saturations at a very small scale. The results show the existence – likely for each phase – of various spatial characteristic scales. Thus the quantitative modelling of the distribution of the various phases implies the identification and the characterization of these characteristic scales. In this paper, we show the existence of a first characteristic scale which allows us to separate properties belonging to the individual packing elements from those belonging to scale of the bed. At this latter scale, heterogeneities still exist. They correspond to spatial correlations which remain to be investigated.

X-ray tomography also allows accurate analysis of the liquid phase distribution. However, liquid films of a few tenths of a millimeter are difficult to detect because their absorbance signal is close to the noise level.

The liquid hold-up values obtained from x-ray tomography measurements seem to be well-represented by a partial wetting model. Therefore one may think that a stochastic approach – as previously proposed [1] – will be needed to model the very intricate distribution of the liquid phase in terms of hydrodynamic properties. Investigations in that direction are currently underway in our laboratory.

6. References

[1]   M. Crine, P. Marchot, and G. L'Homme, AIChE J. **38**:136-47 (1992).

[2]   A. E. Saez, R. G. Carbonell, and J. Levec, AIChE J. **32**:353-68 (1986).

[3]   R. A. Brooks and G. Di Chiro, Phys. Med. Biol. **21**:689-732 (1976).

[4]   A. C. Kak and M. Slaney, Principles of Computerized Tomographic Imaging (IEEE Press, New-York, 1988).

[5]   L. Oger, C. Gauthier, C. Leroy, J. P. Hulin, and E. Guyon, Entropie **25**:29-42 (1989).

[6]   E. T. Jaynes, in R.D. Levine and M. Tribus, editors, The Maximum Entropy Formalism (MIT Press, Cambridge, 1979), p15.

[7]   W. Feller, An Introduction to Probability Theory and Its Application (Wiley, New-York, 1971).

[8]   M. Crine, P. Marchot, B. Lekhlif, and G. L'Homme, Chem.Eng.Sci. **47**:2263-8 (1992).

[9]   B. Lekhlif, Ph.D. Thesis, Université de Liège, Liège (1992).

Appendix

Conference Abstracts

This appendix contains abstracts for papers presented at the Engineering Foundation conference "Frontiers in Industrial Process Tomography", held October 29 through November 3, 1995 at The Cliffs, San Luis Obispo, California. These abstracts will help to complete the overview of process tomography presented in the text, and further information about a particular method or project mentioned in an abstract is available directly from the authors.

The conference has been organized into six principal topics or sessions:

A: Sensor Design
B: Image Reconstruction and Interpretation
C: Environmental Monitoring and Process Control
D: Flow Measurement
E: Separation and Reactor Technology
F: Characterization of Material Structure

The abstracts printed here follow the same order as the conference program and include the keynote addresses, lecture papers, and discussion papers (posters). Post-deadline poster papers are not included.

Session A: Sensor Design

[A.1] Sensor Design and Selection for Single and Multi-Mode Process Tomography

M. S. Beck

Department of Electrical Engineering and Electronics, UMIST, P.O. Box 88, Manchester M60 1QD U.K.

Electrical tomographic sensors using capacitance, conductance, inductance, or microwave techniques offer a modest spatial resolution of about 10%, but they are fast, inexpensive, and suitable for a wide range of vessel sizes. They have been used on mixing vessels, hydrocyclone separators, pneumatic conveyors, oil/gas pipelines, and in imaging the chemi-ionization of flames. These sensors generally distinguish between two phases of components in the object space being interrogated and are classified as single mode sensors. There are many processes where several components exist in the object space and have to be imaged individually. Examples include metallurgical ore separation, coal/shale separation, oil field pipelines, and separators which contain oil, gas, and water. These situations require multi-mode sensing systems.

Multi-mode systems are strictly defined as those in which two or more different sensing entities are used to locate of measure different constituents in the object space. An example of dual mode tomography is taken from the oil industry, where there is a need to measure the quantity of oil, gas, and water in a cross section of an oil well riser. A specific solution uses electrical capacitance tomography for imaging and measuring the water in the oil and ultrasonic tomography for measuring the gas. "Inherently multi-mode systems" are those in which a single imaging method can differentiate between components in the object space.

Electromagnetic tomography is inherently multi-mode and provides an interesting approach to multi-component imaging. It could be particularly useful for metallurgical processes and scrap recycling systems, where ferrous material could be imaged based on its magnetic permeability, and non-ferrous material could be imaged ased on its eddy current loss. Impedance spectroscopy could also be incorporated in the electromagnetic system, which should extend the applicability of this non-contacting echnique.

[A.2] The Physical Basis of Process Tomography

E. J. Morton[1] and S. J. R. Simons[2]

[1] *Department of Physics, University of Surrey, Guildford, Surrey GU2 5XH U.K.*
[2] *Department of Chemical and Biochemical Engineering, University College London, Torrington Place, London WC1E 7JE U.K.*

In recent years many tomographic imaging methods have been developed for possible use within the chemical process industry. However, despite this work, there have been few practical applications of the techniques in industry. It is the focus of this review to attempt to explain why this is so. Resulting from discussions with a number of industrial organizations, an overview of applications important to industry will be presented. This overview will consider not only the type of application, but also the end-use of the system. A review of currently available imaging techniques will be presented to outline the physical constraints on which each technique is based. By combining the information gathered on application areas with the constraints inherent in each technique, suggestions will be made to indicate where we perceive the strengths of process tomography to lie.

[A.3] Optimization of the Operating Frequency in the Design of Microwave Sensors for Projection or Tomographic Inspection

J. Ch. Bolomey

Laboratoire des Signaux et Systèmes, Ecole Supérieure d'Electricité,

Plateau de Moulon, F-91192 Gif-sur-Yvette, Cedex, France

The operating frequency constitutes a factor of prime importance in the performance of microwave sensors devoted to the inspection of industrial materials and processes. First of all, the interaction mechanism between microwave beams and materials is highly sensitive to frequency, due to the frequency dependence of the complex permittivity of materials and hence from the complex propagation constant. Secondly, the operating frequency has a direct impact on the design of the microwave sensor and on the selection of an appropriate wavefront processing technique. In practice, the operating frequency results from a compromise between complexity and performance.

In this paper, the optimization of the operating frequency is analyzed in the light of the most recent advances in the field of inverse scattering theory and non-linear reconstruction algorithms. Compared to more conventional quasi-optical approaches, it is shown that this new point of view results in a significant change of the traditional selection rules for the operating frequency; one can expect drastic improvements in the performance of microwave imaging techniques in the near future. The discussion will be oriented toward industrial applications (such as the control of thin or laminated conveyed products, fluids in pipes, or buried objects) for which microwave sensing is recognized to offer some specific advantages.

[A.4]   Multiple Active Sensors in Ultrasonic Process Tomography Systems

W. Li and B. S. Hoyle

Department of Electronics and Electrical Engineering, University of Leeds, Leeds LS2 9JT   U.K.

In many industrial processes the application of ultrasonic process tomography requires fast data collection. For example, in the on-line measurement of a 2 or 3 component flowing mixture with entrained gas the projections must be obtained in a short enough time interval that the flow evolution is insignificant. Measurement times in ultrasonic systems are intrinsically limited by the speed of sound, which is very low compared with electromagnetic waves.

The paper explores this intrinsic limitation and provides a brief review of parallel data sensor systems, including the use of multiple active receiving sensors and multiple segmented receivers. Results of new investigations of multiple active transmitting sensors are presented which, with suitable encoding, can be shown to offer a significant enhancement to the data acquisition performance of ultrasonic process tomography systems. The paper presents theoretical models for the behavior of a novel Multiple Transmitter Active Concurrently (MTAC) system and then presents a range of simulations of its performance. Conclusions are drawn for the possible exploitation of the method in the industrial application of ultrasonic process tomography.

[A.5]　Stress Tensor Tomography Using Integrated Photoelasticity

A. Trächtler

Institut für Meß- und Regelungstechnik, Universität (T.H.) Karlsruhe,
Postfach 69 80, D-76128 Karlsruhe, Germany

This paper deals with the determination of three-dimensional inhomogeneous stresses from photoelastic measurements by applying tomographic reconstruction methods. A 3-D photoelastic object with spatially varying stress tensor is illuminated by linearly polarized light with variable orientation. In the presence of stresses the object is birefringent, and the photoelastic stress patterns can be seen with an analyzer. For quantitative analysis the stress patterns are recorded by a CCD camera and processed in a computer. In conventional photoelastic measurements one investigates only 2-D stresses orthogonal to the direction of light propagation. Three-dimensional problems are usually treated by freezing the stress and cutting the object into thin slices to approximate a 2-D stress state. In contrast, in integrated photoelasticity 3-D problems are investigated directly; thus the object does not need to be destroyed. With some restrictions (e.g., constancy of the principle axes of the stress tensor on the light ray) the observed birefringence is related to the stress distribution as the line integral over the principle stress difference. For these cases, tomographic methods have been used. For the general case of arbitrary 3-D stresses, the vectorial characterization of polarized light complicates the relation between stress and birefringence, and the tomographic reconstruction problem is non-linear. Thus it would be desirable to have both methods and instruments for experimentally determining arbitrary 3-D stresses.

The first step in photoelastic tomography is to analyze the tomographic mapping to determine which kind of stress fields can be reconstructed in principle. This will be done within a linear approximation using a Fourier transform and the projection slice theorem. Secondly, special efficient reconstruction algorithms are developed. It will be shown that from a methodical point of view photoelastic tomography is somewhere in the middle between linear tomography and diffraction tomography. It is related to non-linear diffraction tomography due to the inhomogeneous and anisotropic optical properties of the object, and it is related to linear tomography as well since the interaction of light with the object can be modeled using geometric optics. This paper will present the new theory and the first experimental results.

[A.6]   The Design of Sensor and Sensor Electronics for a Mutual Inductance Tomography System

A. Peyton
Department of Electrical Engineering and Electronics, UMIST, P.O. Box 88, Manchester M60 1QD U.K.

This paper describes the design and development of a mutual inductance tomography system. The system is capable of imaging the distribution of material which is electrically conductive or magnetic. An optimum design of the sensor is presented, and its fundamental sensitivity limits are discussed and analyzed. The paper also contains a description of the sensor electronics, including a novel base signal compensation scheme. Sample images are presented which point the way forward to possible future industrial applications.

[A.7] Electrical Capacitance Tomography: From Design to Applications

C. G. Xie, W. Q. Wang, and M. S. Beck
*Department of Electrical Engineering and Electronics, UMIST, P.O. Box 88,
Manchester M60 1QD U.K.*

This paper reviews the current status of electrical capacitance tomography (ECT) techniques in the following aspects: transducer and electrode design, image reconstruction and interpretation, process applications, and future development.

The design of highly sensitive capacitance measuring circuits and the associated sensing electrodes are the key to ECT techniques. We discuss two types of capacitance measuring circuits used in process tomography: one based on the charge/discharge principle, and another based on AC phase-sensitive (synchronous detection) techniques. The design of the sensing electrodes is important because the number and size of electrodes are often restricted by the resolution of the capacitance sensing circuits.

Image reconstruction algorithms developed for ECT can be categorized into three groups: backprojection based on a sensitivity matrix, iterative algorithms based on optimization techniques, and methods based on artificial neural networks. The suitability of these approaches are discussed for particular applications.

Process applications of ECT systems are numerous. The following examples will be illustrated:
- tomographic metering of gas/oil/water multiphase flows in pipelines
- transient flows in the blow-off of pressurized vessels
- contact efficiency study in trickle-bed and monolithic reactors
- imaging of gas/solids fluidized beds
- flame propagation in internal combustion engines

[A.8]   New Electronics for a Multi-electrode Electrical Capacitance Tomography System

F. T. Kuhn[1], J. C. Schouten[1], R. F. Mudde[2], P. A. van Halderen[2],
C. M. van den Bleek[1], and B. Scarlett[1]

[1] *Department of Chemical Process Technology, Delft University of Technology,*
   P.O. Box 5, 2600 AA Delft, The Netherlands

[2] *Department of Physical Technology, Delft University of Technology, P.O. Box 5,*
   2600 AA Delft, The Netherlands

It is a known fact that the image resolution of the current electrical tomography systems is relatively poor compared to the other tomographic methods. The main reasons for the low quality of the images by the current 12-electrode electrical capacitance tomography (ECT) systems are first the so-called soft field error due to the neglected dependency of the electrostatic field during the measurement on the still unknown material distribution, and second, the small number of independent measurements per image. One way to enhance the spatial resolution is to increase the number of electrodes mounted around the perimeter of the pipe. This increase, however, leads to a very small electrode surface area and, consequently, to extremely small capacitance values requiring very high-accuracy capacitance transducers.

We are developing a transducer to resolve very small capacitances (under 1 fF) at a high data capture rate, e.g., one frame measured within 0.16 ms when using a 16-electrode sensor. The detection of the capacitance is performed by using the capacitor, which is formed by two of the electrodes and the material between them, as an element of an active differentiator. The input signal of this differentiator is a pulse of constant amplitude with a known rise and fall time. The output signal directly serves as a measure of the capacitance to be determined.

The system sensitivity is enhanced by performing a calibration measurement and using the calibration data as a reference, so the change of the capacitance (relative to an average value) is detected. Furthermore, the use of active differentiators allows for the simultaneous detection of the capacitances of the capacitors formed by one "source" electrode (applied with a high potential) and all the other "detecting" electrodes (kept at zero potential). This capability contributes to the high data capture rate.

[A.9] Design of a Capacitance Tomographic Imaging System with a Rotating Parallel Excitation Field

W. Q. Yang, A. L. Stott, and M. S. Beck

Department of Electrical Engineering and Electronics, UMIST, P.O. Box 88, Manchester M60 1QD U.K.

The existing electrical capacitance tomography (ECT) systems apply an excitation signal to only one of the sensor electrodes at a given time. The electric field produced by single-electrode excitation is not uniform. Consequently the image resolution in the middle is poor compared with that near the wall. To solve this problem, a new 16-electrode ECT system has been designed to produce a rotating parallel excitation field with a uniform capacitance sensitivity distribution. The system hardware consists of AC-based capacitance measuring circuits with feedback compensation to cancel the standing capacitances, a micro-controller, two back-to-back link adaptors for serial communication, and a PC to reconstruct the images. This system can collect measurement data at 100 frames per second, with lower speeds for reconstruction and image display.

[A.10] Simulation Study of the Electrode Array in Electrical Resistance Tomography (ERT)

Fenglan Dong, Yixin Ma, Yongtao Han, and Lingan Xu

Department of Electrical Engineering and Automation, Tianjin University, Tianjin 300072 China

In recent years, the Electrical Resistance Tomography (ERT) technique has been successfully used in several laboratory studies. However, the electrode array's construction (including the shape and dimensions of the electrodes, the driving mode, and the geometry of the array) still needs to be studied in detail. A circular electrode array, for example, has a complicated sensing field with a large sensing volume and an uneven sensitivity distribution, which make the image reconstruction and interpretation difficult.

In order to optimize the array design to get an even sensitivity distribution in the sensing field and to improve the spatial resolution, a finite element method is used to analyze the effects of the electrode shape, size, arrangement, and excitation mode. By comparing simulations with experimental results, several valuable conclusions can be drawn about the design of the electrode array.

[A.11] A Comparison of the Cost for a Magnetic Resonance Imaging Process Sensor with Other Tomographic Techniques

M. J. McCarthy, J. Sanders, and L. Burnett
Department of Food Science and Technology, University of California, Davis, California 95616 U.S.A.

Historically, nuclear magnetic resonance (NMR) and NMR Imaging equipment have been characterized as extremely costly. While this is true for medical whole body imaging and very high magnetic field research systems, this has not been the case for low field permanent magnet based instruments. For most applications in process monitoring the requirements for nuclear magnetic resonance are such that low field permanent magnets or electromagnets are the appropriate technology. These systems would additionally be designed for a single type of measurement, resulting in more cost savings. For most process tomography applications, this will result in an NMR based system which is cost competitive with other process tomography modalities. Several case studies will be presented that demonstrate the costs of NMR based process sensors.

[A.12]   Simulation of Electric Field Distribution in a Micro-tomographic System

T. M. Shi[1], R. A. Williams[2], M. Wang[3], F. J. Dickin[3], C. G. Xie[3], and M. S. Beck[3]

[1] *Department of Chemical Engineering, UMIST, Manchester M60 1QD U.K.*

[2] *Camborne School of Mines, University of Exeter, Redruth, Cornwall TR15 3SE U.K.*

[3] *Department of Electrical Engineering and Electronics, UMIST, Manchester M60 1QD U.K.*

The effects of interactions between electrodes that are closely placed around the inside wall of the transporting tube are simulated via a finite element model. Because the simulation is aimed at optimizing micro-tomographic imaging (for example, mapping emulsion droplets in either an oil-in-water or a water-in-oil state), it is conducted under three conditions:

(1) in a homogeneous medium with different electrical impedance properties;

(2) in an oil-in-water emulsion at constant concentration; and

(3) in a water-in-oil emulsion at constant concentration.

The comparison of different sensitivity maps will be made and suggestions about measurement procedure and instrument design will be given.

Session B: Image Reconstruction and Interpretation

[B.1]   Sensing Principles, Types of Interactions, and Their Impact on Reconstruction

F. Mesch

Institut für Meß- und Regelungstechnik, Universität (T.H.) Karlsruhe, Postfach 69 80, D-76128 Karlsruhe, Germany

The original paper by Radon dealt with line integrals along parallel, straight integration paths; the Radon transform and its inverse were later found to be an adequate model and mathematical tool for computerized tomography when first applied to x-rays in medicine. The subsequent meteoric development of tomography in medicine and more recently for process applications has included many other physical principles for sensing.

Whereas the interaction of x-rays with tissue is absorption, the newer physical principles exhibit quite different types of interaction, described by more complex mathematical models, and thus require different reconstruction algorithms.

In this paper, various types of interaction are reviewed and systemically classified. Classification is done first into scalar , vectorial, and tensorial interaction. Examples of scalar interactions are absorption, reflection, scattering, or impedance; examples of vectorial interactions are velocity and refractive index fields measured by ultrasonics or optics, and tensorial interactions occur in measuring stress fields. Another criterion for classification is the type of integrals involved; line integrals (along either straight or curved paths), volume integrals, and general integral equations occur. Based on this classification, some general statements and rules regarding the design of sensor arrays and the obtainable spatial resolution are given. These general statements are illustrated by examples and typical applications in process tomography.

[B.2]   Reconstruction Enhancement for Electrical Capacitance Tomography

N. Reinecke and D. Mewes

Institut für Verfahrenstechnik, Universität Hannover, Callinstraße 36
D-30167 Hannover, Germany

Normally, the reconstruction of images in capacitance tomography is done using simple backward solving algorithms such as backprojection. This is a crude simplification because only the forward problem is immediately solvable. Therefore, an iterative algorithm for the non-linear capacitance tomography was developed. This algebraic reconstruction technique (ART) is already widely used in linear tomography, for example holographic interferometry or any other optical tomography. For the reconstruction of the set of non-linear measurements, a linearization of the electric field problem was conducted. This linearization is not necessary for the iterative loop, but it increases the speed of the reconstruction by orders of magnitude compared to the direct forward solution utilizing a finite element approach. In the paper it is shown that different optimization strategies in the correction affect the convergence and reconstruction quality of the algorithm.

Using measurements conducted with capacitance sensors, a dynamic correction of the data is introduced. In electrical tomography the measurements have to be taken sequentially to avoid interference from the developing field. For slow processes this restriction does not affect the reconstruction. For transient processes, though, the reconstruction quality can be enhanced by interpolating the measurements. This greatly reduces the blur due to the delay between subsequent measurements. A cubic steady spline with two steady derivatives at the actual measurement points was used for the interpolation. From simulated results the paper shows the maximum velocity of the measured structures that can be allowed without observing aliased images.

[B.3] Performance of Neural Networks for Image Reconstruction and Interpretation in ECT Process Tomography Systems

A. Y. Nooralahiyan, B. S. Hoyle, and N. J. Bailey
Department of Electronics and Electrical Engineering, University of Leeds,
Leeds LS2 9JT U.K.

Electrical Capacitance Tomography (ECT) is a well researched technique for non-invasive measurement potentially applicable to a wide range of industrial applications. Its spatial resolution is limited by the number of capacitance electrodes, which in turn governs the computational needs of the conventional linear back-projection image reconstruction algorithm. For systems with relatively fast dynamics (such as the flow in an oil field pipeline) intensive processing is required, typically demanding a parallel computer solution. In contrast, a trained artificial neural network has been shown by the authors to provide an efficient alternative. The paper presents results from this research program on the flexibility and interpolation of such networks under noise variations for simulated oil field pipeline data. It also illustrates the feasibility of training a single network to reconstruct images in water-continuous as well as oil-continuous situations, without the need for recalibration.

A multi-output network is used as a pattern associator to provide the cross-sectional image and to allow the on-line estimation of component fractions. A following classifying network is a multilayer perceptron trained to identify four different flow regimes: stratified, bubble, core, and annular flow. Examples presented are based on training sets which consist of the smallest identifiable elements of high permittivity (water droplets) placed in different positions within the low permittivity component (oil) and *vice versa* . The same network is trained for oil continuous and water continuous flows, and the combined training sets cover the entire cross section of the pipe. Two networks have been trained for components with a large difference in permittivity (oil/water) and a small difference in permittivity (oil/gas), with comparable results. The results for image reconstruction, interpretation, and tolerance to noise are fully illustrated. The paper concludes with suggestions for industrial exploitation of the technique.

[B.4]   Test of a Model-Based Reconstruction Algorithm for Quantitative Reconstruction of Process Tomography Data

Ø. Isaksen[1], B. T. Hjertaker[2], A. S. Dico[1,2]

[1] *Chr. Michelsen Research, Fantoft vg. 38, N-5036 Fantoft, Norway*

[2] *Department of Physics, University of Bergen, Allegaten 55, N-5007 Bergen, Norway*

Reconstruction of process tomography data is often based on a small number of measurements, which may in addition suffer from soft-field effects. This means that powerful reconstruction techniques developed for medical tomography cannot be used for a process tomography system. At the University of Bergen and Chr. Michelsen Research there has been developed a new reconstruction algorithm called Model-Based Reconstruction (MOR). The algorithm is based on minimizing the difference between measurements and simulated measurements which are based on the medium distribution inside the cross-section. The distribution of the medium is given as input to a model of the sensor system which calculates the simulated measurements. The distribution is then changed in an iterative scheme so that the difference between the measured and simulated measurements converge towards a minimum. This algorithm has been tested for imaging separation processes and pipe flow, and the results show that MOR represents a step towards quantitative process tomography. In this paper the principle of the MOR algorithm will be outlined, and test results will be presented.

[B.5]   Improving Image Reconstruction of Field Electrical Resistance Tomography Data

A. Binley[1], A. Ramirez[2], and W. Daily[2]

[1] CRES, *Institute of Environmental and Biological Sciences, Lancaster University,*
Lancaster LA1 4YQ U.K.

[2] *Lawrence Livermore National Laboratory, P.O. Box 808, Livermore,*
California 94550 U.S.A.

Cross borehole electrical resistance tomography (ERT) is capable of providing detailed information of the spatial structure of subsurface resistivity. This can benefit assessments of ground water contamination and hydrogeological and geotechnical site characterization. In addition this new geophysical tool is capable, in many cases, of providing a monitoring process for ground water decontamination or remediation and thus has great value in the current climate of environmental concern.

Various measurement schemes have been proposed for cross borehole ERT. Given that field data is often flawed with errors, one of the principal aims here is to examine the role of data error on various measurement schemes. Although this has been attempted in previous studies using synthetic data, the research here focuses on actual field data from a well-characterized site. In addition, an examination is made of new ideas for improving image reconstruction in cases where *a priori* information is available. In this case, focus is made on the use of geological data in conditioning the inverse methods for ERT; however, the conclusions may be generally applicable to a variety of tomographic imaging methods.

[B.6]   An X-Ray CT Reconstruction Algorithm for Industrial Applications

A. B. Cortes, C. L. Lin, and J. D. Miller
Department of Metallurgical Engineering, University of Utah, Salt Lake City, Utah 84112 U.S.A.

X-ray computed tomography (CT) is an excellent tool for studying the internal structure and texture of multiphase materials in a non-invasive and nondestructive manner. In order to utilize x-ray CT as a quantitative tool in industrial applications, the amount of reconstruction error must be minimized. Reconstruction algorithms derived from the medical field exhibit large errors in the presence of high-density materials. To correct this deficiency, an iterative reconstruction algorithm is introduced which reduces the reconstruction error significantly. Simulation results using this new reconstruction algorithm are presented.

[B.7]   Direct   Algebraic   Reconstruction   in   Electromagnetic Flow Tomography

A. Wernsdörfer

Institut für Meß- und Regelungstechnik, Universität (T.H.) Karlsruhe, Postfach 69 80, D-76128 Karlsruhe, Germany

Electromagnetic flow measurement has many applications due to its accuracy and non-invasive measuring principle. The voltage induced by an external exciting magnetic field and measured by a pair of electrodes is proportional to the mean velocity of the fluid, provided the flow profile is circularly symmetric. If this condition is not fulfilled, the meter gives erroneous results. In such cases the determination of the local distribution by tomography would enable the measurement of the flow rate independent of the profile. Up to now a series expansion method was utilized to solve the inverse problem of calculating the local distribution of flow velocity from the volume integrals making up the measurement. This approach leads to a large number of unknowns, and the resulting set of equations is ill-conditioned, which causes distortions due to noisy data.

In this paper a new reconstruction method is adapted to the problem. As proven in other applications, the so-called Direct Algebraic Reconstruction (DAR) yields extraordinarily good results compared to other methods, particularly if the amount of data is small. The main reason for this good performance is a measurement model which closely approximates reality. The adaptation of DAR to electromagnetic flow tomography and the reconstruction of the flow field are discussed. A very efficient implementation is proposed which yields a high reconstruction speed. The superiority of this method is demonstrated by reconstructing arbitrary flow profiles from data measured in an existing experimental set-up.

[B.8]   The Effect of Measurement Noise on Numerical Reconstruction Algorithms for EIT

J. A. Dell and J. Artola

Department of Electronics, University of York, Heslington, York YO1 5DD U.K.

This paper outlines a series of numerical experiments with simulated electrical impedance tomographic (EIT) data and various levels of additive Gaussian noise. The properties of well-known finite element reconstruction algorithms employing such techniques as singular value decomposition (SVD) and QR factorization are examined. Practical results which clearly show the performance degradation caused by noise are provided, and the mathematical basis for the conclusions are discussed.

[B.9]   An On-line Ultrasound Tomography System: Implementation and Its Application

Lingan Xu and Lijun Xu
Department of Electrical Engineering and Automation, Tianjin University,
Tianjin 300072 China

On the basis of analyzing the propagation of ultrasound through a bubbly gas/liquid two-phase flow (which is considered to be a strongly inhomogeneous medium due to the high contrast in acoustic impedance distribution), a transmission mode (TM) Ultrasound Computerized Tomography (UCT) system was developed. In order to speed the data acquisition and image reconstruction, a parallel processing design of both hardware and software was adopted in this system. When this system was used for monitoring the movement of a bubble (or multi-bubble group) rising from the bottom of a static liquid column, the reconstructed image showed that its real-time performance was fairly good.

In this paper, the parallel design and real-time sector logic back-projection reconstruction algorithm are described. Two methods (the area method and the barycenter method) are introduced to analyze the quality of the reconstructed image. Furthermore, criteria that measure the real-time performance of this system are discussed. Some experimental results are given as well. Finally, the application of UCT to monitoring a two-phase flow is discussed.

[B.10]   Electrodynamic Sensors for Process Tomography

R. G. Green, K. Evans, A. Goude, M. Henry, and M. E. Shackelton
School of EIT, Sheffield Hallam University, Pond Street, Sheffield S1 1WB U.K.

Many industrial processes use pneumatic conveying of dry particulates in the manufacturing process (e.g., pulverized fuel in cement manufacture). Measurement of the volume or mass flow rate of dry particulates can improve the control and the efficiency of the manufacturing system. Measurement in pneumatic conveyors is often difficult because the solids, conveyed at high Reynolds number, are not evenly distributed within a cross section of the conveyor. In traveling through the conveyor the solids will usually obtain an electrostatic charge. This charge is a function of the material conveyed, conveyor construction, particle size and shape, and humidity. However, our tests indicate that the electrical charge produced is statistically constant for specific processes.

This electrical charge may be measured using an electrodynamic transducer, which consists of a rugged, low cost sensing electrode into which the flowing charged particles induce charge, followed by a charge-to-voltage converter. An array consisting of several identical devices may be used to measure the volume flow rate of pneumatically conveyed solids by producing a tomographic image of the concentration of material in a cross section of the flow pipe and integrating these concentrations with respect to time.

A difficulty with producing concentration images using electrodynamic sensors is that the reconstruction algorithms, which convert the measured data into a concentration profile, are dependent on the initial distribution of solids in the sensing volume, i.e., the flow regime. If the flow regime is known, the reconstruction may be simplified and speeded up. The flow regime can be recognized by a suitably organized and trained neural network. This paper describes a tomographic imaging system that uses electrodynamic sensors and a neural network to identify the flow regime and select the appropriate reconstruction algorithm.

[B.11] Tomographic Imaging of Transparent Slurries with Particle Sizing Using Optical Fibers

N. M. Horbury[1], R. A. Rahim[1,2], F. J. Dickin[3], R. G. Green[1], B. D. Naylor[1], and T. P. Pridmore[1]

[1] *School of EIT, Sheffield Hallam University, Pond Street, Sheffield S1 1WB U.K.*

[2] *Faculty of Electrical Engineering, University Teknologi, Malaysia*

[3] *Department of Electrical Engineering and Electronics, UMIST, Manchester M60 1QD U.K.*

Process tomography provides non-intrusive methods of viewing cross sections of a process. The method presented here is used to investigate solid particles being hydraulically transported. Optical fibers are used as guides to carry light to and from the measurement section. Each transmitter/receiver pair of fibers provides a single "view", in which the intensity of light falling upon the receiving fiber is modulated by the presence of an object in its path. The modulated light signal is converted into an analog electrical signal, which is then digitized for computer analysis. Using computational methods and several projections, an image of the process can be formed. The use of small diameter optical fibers allows many "views" per projection and thus permit a high spatial resolution to be achieved. Analysis is also being carried out on the frequency component of the received light levels to investigate the information content relating to the size of the particles in the process. Combining this information with the image of the process will give flow profiles of both solids concentration and size distribution. Work has been carried out using particles in the range of 100 - 600 microns; thus range is now being extended upwards.

[B.12]   Tomographic Imaging System Using Optical Fibers for Pneumatic Conveyors

R. A. Rahim[1,2], N. M. Horbury[1], F. J. Dickin[3], R. G. Green[1], B. D. Naylor[1], and T. P. Pridmore[1]

[1] *School of EIT, Sheffield Hallam University, Pond Street, Sheffield S1 1WB U.K.*
[2] *Faculty of Electrical Engineering, University Teknologi, Malaysia*
[3] *Department of Electrical Engineering and Electronics, UMIST, Manchester M60 1QD*
     U.K.

This paper describes the initial work which has been completed on a tomographic imaging system using optical fiber sensors for application to pneumatically conveyed solids. The overall aim of the project is to produce tomographic images relating to particle size distribution and concentration distribution over the cross section of the measurement section. The system under development uses an array of 32 transducer pairs, aligned in a square matrix.

Practical tests have been carried out on a prototype system built into a metal pipe of 100 mm diameter. The present illumination system uses a single quartz halogen light source coupled to the optical transmitter fibers, which are arranged in a bundle. The light arriving at the receiver fibers is modulated by the flowing solids and converted to an electrical signal by PIN diodes. The transducer is surrounded by a grounded screen to minimize the effects of electrical and optical noise. The output is amplified and conditioned for the data capture system.

A series of experiments have been carried out which investigate the effects of particle size and concentration on the received signals. The particle sizes range from 100 microns to 2 mm.

Session C: Environmental Monitoring and Process Control

[C.1]   Detecting Leaks from Underground Tanks Using Electrical Resistance Tomography

A. Ramirez[1], W. Daily[1], D. LaBrecque[2], A. Binley[3]

[1] *Lawrence Livermore National Laboratory, P.O. Box 808, Livermore,*
    California 94550 U.S.A.

[2] *University of Arizona, Tucson, Arizona 85721 U.S.A.*

[3] *University of Lancaster, Lancaster LA1 4YQ U.K.*

Leaks from underground storage tanks account for contamination of soil and ground water world-wide. A method is needed to detect the presence and location of such leaks to assist in soil clean-up. We are investigating the use of electrical resistance tomography (ERT) to locate leaks from buried steel tanks. The reconstruction is based on a regularized iterative Newton type equation. Because the tank contents are very electrically conductive, a plume will be detected as a change in resistivity in the reconstructed image. We have completed the first phase of a test in which 1040 gallons of water were released. Images before and after the release show a clear anomaly of decreasing electrical resistivity beneath the tank, centered on the release point. This anomaly is noticeable after release of only 100 gallons of water. The electrical contrast and lateral extent of the anomaly grow during the course of the release and then decrease after the release is terminated.

[C.2]   Applications of Crosshole Seismic Tomography at Environmental Sites

G. L. Elbring

Geophysics Department 6116, Sandia National Laboratories, P.O. Box 5800, Albuquerque, New Mexico 87185-0750 U.S.A.

In the testing and remediation of environmental sites, good information on the subsurface is required to model hydrogeologic processes, place wells, and choose the best remediation effort. In the past this characterization has been done through well logs and well sampling. As regions increase in complexity, point samples from wells have proved to be inadequate to map the subsurface. The role of crosshole seismic imaging is to fill in the geologic information between the boreholes in terms of both lithology and saturation characteristics.

A number of borehole seismic sources have been used over the course of these experiments. These have generated energy primarily in the lower frequencies (30 Hz to 500 Hz) and are able to penetrate the unconsolidated near surfaces to distances on the order of 100 meters. Spatial resolution for these frequencies is on the order of 1 - 3 meters for these types of sites. Both compressional and shear waves are generated and analyzed. The variation in sensitivity of these two wave types to fluid content aids in the interpretation of saturation level in the formations.

Several surveys have been carried out at DOE sites to determine the efficacy and capabilities of this imaging technique. These have been conducted in the near-surface (within 100 meters) in formations including both alternating sand and clay sequences and alternating sand and gravel sequences. Surveys have encompassed regions both above the water table (where coupling of the seismic energy is less efficient) and below the water table. The surveys have been successful not only in imaging the geologic sequence but also in providing information on variations in soil saturation due to both natural (perched water zones) and man-made (vapor stripping remediation) causes.

[C.3]   Design and Control of Slurry Mixing Processes Using Electrical Resistance Tomography

R. A. Williams[1], X. Jia[2], F. J. Dickin[2], S. L. McKee[3], and A. Boxman[4]

[1] *Camborne School of Mines, University of Exeter, Redruth, Cornwall TR15 3SE U.K.*

[2] *Department of Electrical Engineering and Electronics, UMIST, P.O. Box 88, Manchester M60 1QD U.K.*

[3] *Department of Chemical Engineering, UMIST, P.O. Box 88, Manchester M60 1QD U.K.*

[4] *Du Pont Central Research and Development, Du Pont Company, P.O. Box 80304, Wilmington, Delaware 19880-0304 U.S.A.*

The recent development of rapid tomographic imaging methods based on electrical sensors offers a powerful means to monitor and control process mixing and dispersion. During the last three years a data bank of experimental measurements of the concentration distributions within agitated solid-liquid mixers has been acquired using a pseudo-three-dimensional electrical resistance imaging method.

The technique involves placing a ring of 16 or more electrodes on the inner wall of the mixing vessel. A small AC excitation current is injected into each electrode sequentially, while monitoring the electrical potential generated at all other (passive) electrodes. These data are used to solve the Laplace equation to reconstruct the two-dimensional conductivity distribution within the cross section. The solids concentration is then predicted from the measured conductivities based on an empirical (Maxwell-type) correlation for the solid-liquid mixture under investigation. By installing a number of electrode planes on the mixer it is possible to make measurements at multiple cross-sections and hence characterize the entire volume of the vessel.

This contribution will demonstrate how tomographic information can be used: to monitor the mixing efficiency, to provide data for development of empirical models for the design of mixer geometry, to investigate the effects of particle size distribution on mixing behavior, to provide data to validate and develop theoretical fluid dynamics models, and to control batch solid-liquid and liquid-liquid mixing processes. Other important opportunities for using electrical resistance tomography to monitor and control particle transport (conveying) and separation processes will be reviewed.

[C.4] Monitoring and Control of Powder Flow Using Capacitance Tomography

R. B. Edwards[1], T. Dyakowski[2], C. G. Xie[3], and R. A. Williams[4]

[1] *Unilever Research Port Sunlight Laboratory, Quarry Road East, Bebington, Wirral L63 3JW U.K.*

[2] *Department of Chemical Engineering, UMIST, P.O. Box 88, Manchester M60 1QD U.K.*

[3] *Schlumberger Cambridge Research, High Cross, Madingley Road, Cambridge CB3 0EL U.K.*

[4] *Camborne School of Mines, University of Exeter, Redruth, Cornwall TR15 3SE U.K.*

The aim of this case study is to present the results of an industrial application of capacitance tomography to investigate solid distribution within a chute in an operating plant. Chutes are commonly used in many chemical and food plants to convey solids between various heat or mass transfer apparatus. Steady state and homogeneous solid distribution is assumed at the inlet cross-section to the heat or mass transfer exchangers. On the other hand, solids are fed into the chute by various types of feeders, including rotary feeders. Such feeders inevitably generate some kind of pulsation which causes the solid distribution to be both non-stationary and non-homogeneous. Therefore the real flow conditions are different from the assumed ones. The difference between ideal and non-ideal conditions can be characterized by the solid distribution pattern at the chute cross-section.

To investigate solid distribution within the chute, a 12-electrode capacitance tomography system has been applied in an operating industrial plant. Solid particles with diameter in the range of 14 - 200 microns and a density of 2400 kg-m^3 were conveyed within the chute. The 12 sensor electrodes were mounted on the outer surface of the chute. The 66 independent measured capacitive values were sent to the transputer network via an optical link for image reconstruction. The images were reconstructed using a qualitative filtered linear backprojection algorithm. The results show that this system is capable of monitoring fine solids with concentrations larger than 5%. A correlation is shown between the movement of the solids and the periodicity caused by the rotary feeder. Future process control and monitoring applications are discussed.

[C.5]   Use of Electrical Impedance Tomography for Controlling Hydrocyclone Underflow Discharge

J. A. Gutiérrez[1], T. Dyakowski[2], M. S. Beck[1], and R. A. Williams[3]

[1] *Department of Electrical Engineering and Electronics, UMIST, P.O. Box 88, Manchester M60 1QD U.K.*

[2] *Department of Chemical Engineering, UMIST, P.O. Box 88, Manchester M60 1QD U.K.*

[3] *Camborne School of Mines, University of Exeter, Redruth, Cornwall TR15 3SE U.K.*

The control of mineral processing plants may be improved by using tomographic techniques to measure the quantity and spatial distribution of materials at certain points in the process. Particularly for solid-liquid separation, where it is difficult even to measure the input and output streams, a tomographic imaging system could provide an economical solution for multiflow measurement. Electrical Impedance Tomography (EIT) can provide real-time data capture (over 200 frames per second based on 16 electrodes and current injection at 100 kHz), suggesting that rapid fluctuations in concentration can be examined. Thus, measurement at a critical point in the process could be used in a feedback control scheme to give reliable and safe operation at maximum throughput. In addition, tomographic images can provide data for model verification procedures that could result in improved models of process behavior.

The results of a series of experiments using EIT to investigate multi-phase flow characteristics will be presented. Images were reconstructed using *qualitative* and *quantitative* image reconstruction algorithms. The resulting tomograms can provide useful information on various aspects of hydrocyclone performance. The air core can also be observed, and its size and position relative to the center of the separator can be measured. In addition, the effect of feed flow rate and particle concentration over the separation process can be determined.

[C.6]   The Role of Process Tomography in Process Control

S. J. R. Simons

Department of Chemical and Biochemical Engineering, University College London, Torrington Place, London WC1E 7JE U.K.

The technique of process tomography has recently been advanced as having an application in process control. Whilst other techniques are already well established in this field (e.g., acoustic pyrometers, gamma-ray densitometers and level probes, and ultrasonic flow meters), process tomography is still at an early stage of development and is yet to find a particular niche which will enable it to supersede conventional control instrumentation.

In this paper, an overview of the benefits to be gained from advanced instrument-based process control systems is given, and the role that process tomography may play in such systems is discussed. Particular areas for exploitation of the technique are put forward and suggestions are made as to how this exploitation could be achieved.

[C.7]   Electrical Resistance Tomography Imaging of Ionic Transport through Soil in an Electric Field

L. J. West[1], D. I. Stewart[2], A. M. Bailey[3], and B. C. B. Shaw[3]

[1] *Department of Earth Sciences, University of Leeds, Leeds LS2 9JT U.K.*

[2] *Department of Civil Engineering, University of Leeds, Leeds LS2 9JT U.K.*

[3] *CRES, Institute of Environmental and Biological Sciences, Lancaster University, Lancaster LA1 4YQ U.K.*

Electrokinetic treatment is a developing technology for treating contaminated land. An electric current (of the order of 0.5 A/m^2) is passed through the soil, causing migration of charged species towards collection wells. In fine grained soils pore water flow is also induced. Many laboratory studies have been carried out to characterize electrokinetic transport. However, these have relied upon destructive analysis of specimens. Here, electrical resistance tomography (ERT) is used to monitor changes of resistivity in a soil specimen during electrokinetic treatment.

Cylindrical specimens of reconstituted Speswhite kaolinite loaded with 1000 ppm of lead nitrate were subjected to an electrical potential gradient of 37.5 V/m. A switched D.C. ERT data acquisition system was used to monitor the spatial variation of sample resistivity. Quantitative images were reconstructed of both transverse and longitudinal sections of the specimen during decontamination. Specimens were sectioned and analyzed for pH and lead concentration after testing, to permit correlation of resistivity changes with the chemical conditions.

The images presented show a region of relatively low resistivity develops near the anode and progresses towards the cathode. This is due to acid, produced by electrolysis at the anode, entering the specimen and reducing the pH from 4 to below 3. In previous studies, radial homogeneity has been assumed. However, the ERT images presented here show that the acid front progression is more rapid in the center of the specimen than around the circumference.

[C.8]   Electrical Resistance Tomography to Image a Subsurface Gasoline Plume

W. Daily[1], A. Ramirez[1], D. LaBrecque[2]

[1] *Lawrence Livermore National Laboratory, P.O. Box 808, Livermore, California 94550 U.S.A.*

[2] *University of Arizona, Tucson, Arizona 85721 U.S.A.*

A controlled experiment was conducted at the Oregon Graduate Institute (OGI) with the purpose of evaluating electrical resistance tomography for imaging free product gasoline in the subsurface. The OGI facilities are unique: a double-wall tank 10 m square and 5 m deep, filled with river bottom sediments and instrumented for geophysical and hydrological studies. This facility allowed us to release a hydrocarbon contaminant into the soil, at a scale sufficiently large to see real-world physical phenomena.

Images of electrical resistivity were made before and during a controlled spill of gasoline into a sandy soil. The primary purpose was to determine if the electrical resistivity images could be used to detect separate phase hydrocarbon in either the vadose or saturated zone. We saw in the tomograms definite changes of electrical resistivity in both the vadose and saturated soils. These effects were an increase in resistivity of as much as 10% above pre-release values. A single resistive anomaly was imaged, directly below the release point, predominately within the vadose zone but extending below the phreatic surface. The anomaly remained identifiable in the tomograms two days after the release ended, with clear indications of lateral spreading along the saturated surface.

Session D: Flow Measurement

[D.1]   Electrical Capacitance Tomography for Fluidized Bed Analysis

T. Dyakowski

Department of Chemical Engineering, UMIST, P.O. Box 88, Manchester M60 1QD U.K.

A knowledge of unsteady solid concentration is vital to characterize the dynamic behavior of a fluidized bed. The flow pattern is determined by particle-particle and particle-gas interactions and bubble coalescence. These interactions, in the time domain, can be characterized by both large and small scale fluctuations. The rapid fluctuations (over intervals of milliseconds or less) of voidage in the bed negate the possibility of using radiation-based sensors, but such phenomena can be sensed using electrical methods.

This paper describes the use of a capacitance tomography (ECT) system for imaging gas bubbles in a fluidized bed . The results show how the solid concentration distribution varies as a function of time for three different flow regimes: bubbling, slugging, and transition to turbulence. Bubble shape, length, and coalescence can be observed. A method of spatial correlation to elucidate the bubble formation process is described. The ECT system can provide a substantial amount of data on the temporal and spatial variations in bed voidage; by applying deterministic chaos theory to this data, one can construct a model for simulating the dynamic behavior of a fluidized bed.

[D.2]   Flow Velocity Tomography with Magnetic Flowmeter

S. Honda, T. Teshima, and Y. Tomita
Faculty of Science and Technology, Keio University, Hiyoshi 3-4-1, Kohoku, Yokohama 223 Japan

Magnetic flowmeters, which have been one of the standard instruments to measure liquid flowrate in industry, were applied to tomographic imaging of a flow velocity field, based on the fact that there are no exciting magnetic fields that induce the flow signal proportional to volumetric flowrate free from the flow profile. The two-dimensional case was examined theoretically for the reason of simplicity, and a flowmeter with eight magnetic poles and eight signal pick-up electrodes was developed. A driving alternating current of one ampere was fed to eight pole pairs and the induced currents were picked up across eight other pairs of electrodes. Flow in the pipe was assumed to be fully developed and axially symmetric. Since the field interaction model of the flowmeter is ill-posed, some prior knowledge (such as the non-negativeness and smoothness of the profile) was introduced to reconstruct the flow field. As a result, when the pipe was moved perpendicularly to its axis, the same reconstruction image was observed. The flowrate estimated with the present equipment agrees with a standard commercially available magnetic flowmeter.

[D.3]   Initial Test of a Dual Mode Tomography for Three-Component Flow Imaging

G. A. Johansen[1,2], Ø. Isaksen[2], T. Frøystein[1], B. T. Hjertaker[1], Ø. Olsen[1], and E. A. Hammer[1,2]

[1] *Department of Physics, University of Bergen, Allegaten 55, N-5007 Bergen, Norway*

[2] *Chr. Michelsen Research, Fantoft vg. 38, N-5036 Fantoft, Norway*

At the University of Bergen (UoB) and Chr. Michelsen Research (CMR) a capacitance tomography and a gamma-ray tomograph have been built and tested for different applications. The capacitance tomography consists of 8 electrodes, a data acquisition system, high sensitivity capacitance detectors, and a reconstruction unit. This system has successfully been tested for pipe flow imaging at Norsk Hydro, CMR, and UoB. It has also been tested for hydrocyclone imaging and three-phase gravity separator imaging at CMR. The gamma-ray tomograph consists of 5 gamma-ray sources and 85 detectors, and it has successfully been tested for pipe flow imaging. In this paper a short description of the system and some test results will be given. The gamma-ray and capacitance systems will also be used as components in a dual mode tomograph for imaging water/oil/gas flow in pipes; some initial results from those tests will also be given.

[D.4]   Comparisons of MRI Velocimetry with Computational Fluid Dynamics

B. Newling[1], S. J. Gibbs[1], L. D. Hall[1], S. Ablett[2], W. Frith[2], and D. E. Haycock[2]

[1] *Herchel Smith Laboratory, Cambridge University School of Clinical Medicine,*
University Forvie Site, Robinson Way, Cambridge CB2 2PZ U.K.
[2] *Unilever Research Laboratories, Colworth House, Sharnbrook,*
Bedfordshire MK44 1LQ U.K.

Magnetic Resonance Imaging (MRI) has considerable potential as a non-invasive method for the study of optically opaque, proton-rich systems. The array of techniques which allow the visualization of fluid flow are of relevance to process engineering.

The particular strength of MRI lies in the variety of physical parameters which may be reflected in the image contrast, dependent upon the specific experimental procedure adopted. We illustrate the use of MRI to obtain a qualitative picture of steady fluid flow and the quantification of that fluid flow by the imposition of motion dependent contrast. In combination with fast imaging techniques (echo planar and FLASH imaging) and Bayesian data analysis, data is provided for construction of three-dimensional velocity maps of fluid flow in a variety of systems. The quantification of fluid velocities permits direct comparison with computational fluid dynamics results for complex geometries of interest and different fluids.

The poster contains details of the implementation of DANTE tagging and pulsed gradient, phase-contrast motion imaging in flowing systems from centimeters to tens of centimeters in size. A two-dimensional acquisition takes only 100 ms and three-dimensional phase contrast images can be acquired in about 30 minutes. Velocity maps of the flow of Newtonian and non-Newtonian fluids in an expansion-contraction model system are compared with computational fluid dynamics results. We consider flow rates from several centimeters per second to half a meter per second.

[D.5]   Measurement of Dispersion Coefficients

C. J. Grootveld, K. J. Bloos, and B. Scarlett
Delft University of Technology, Faculty of Chemical Engineering,
Julianalaan 136 2628 BL Delft, The Netherlands

For the design of hydraulic transport systems it is of the utmost importance to understand fully the solid/liquid flow. Traditionally the design is based on empirical relations for specific problems. However, a more general approach is wanted to solve any hydraulic problem.

The settling dispersion model, which assumes a dynamic equilibrium between the gravitational settling of particles and the dispersion from high to low concentrations, is used to describe the process. The governing equation is known as the convection-dispersion equation, in which the dispersion tensor is a function of local conditions. Therefore a measurement setup is required which accounts for those conditions.

The setup consists of two concentric pipes both carrying slurries with the same velocity and concentration. At the end of the inner pipe the slurries join and at this point the first cross sectional concentration profile is measured. Next the profile is measured at some distance from the injection point. The measurements are then fitted to a known dispersion curve to calculate the dispersion tensor. The measurement technique used is electrical resistance tomography, which enables cross sectional imaging of the concentration.

[D.6]   Electrical Capacitance Tomography Applied to a Fluidized Bed for Spatio-Temporal Chaos Analysis

F. T. Kuhn[1], J. C. Schouten[1], R. F. Mudde[2], C. M. van den Bleek[1], and B. Scarlett[1]

[1] *Department of Chemical Process Technology, Delft University of Technology,*
     P.O. Box 5, 2600 AA Delft, The Netherlands

[2] *Department of Physical Technology, Delft University of Technology, P.O. Box 5,*
     2600 AA Delft, The Netherlands

Up to now, scale-up rules for fluidized beds often fail in practice since they do not account for the time-dependence and non-linearity of the hydrodynamics causing a chaotic system behavior. It is envisaged that the inclusion of the chaotic characteristics of the fluidized beds' hydrodynamics will enhance scale-up procedures. So far, data analysis techniques for non-linear systems have been applied to time series of pressure fluctuations to quantify the chaotic behavior at different flow regimes. The dynamic system behavior is quantified in terms of a) correlation dimension, corresponding to the degrees of freedom and the system's complexity, and b) Kolmogorov entropy, being a measure of the system's time-dependency and short-term predictability. Both invariants enable the hydrodynamic behavior to be related to operational parameters such as gas velocity, aspect ratio, and bed size.

In this paper, we report about a 12-electrode electrical capacitance tomography system applied to a 284 mm ID fluidized bed to record voidage data for small volumes within the bed, to investigate the radial dependency of dimension and entropy on operation parameters. This sensor allows us to relate the bubble dynamics to the overall bed behavior, which is of great use in understanding regime transitions and scale effects.

[D.7] Real-Time Acoustic Planar Imaging of Dense Slurries (RAPIDS)

B. B. Breden[1], R. Shekarriz[1], and H. K. Kytömaa[2]

[1] *Pacific Northwest Laboratory, Richland, Washington U.S.A*

[2] *Failure Analysis Associates, 3 Speen Street, Framingham, Massachusetts 01701 U.S.A.*

An ultrasonic imaging technique is used to measure the velocity and concentration within a solid-liquid slurry. This technique is deemed suitable for non-intrusive quantitative visualization of the flow of an opaque mixture or a flow bounded within opaque walls. Flow of fiber suspensions, polymer melts, and colloidal dispersions are examples of opaque mixtures in which the use of intrusive techniques is not desirable.

Real-Time Acoustic Planar Imaging of Dense Slurries (RAPIDS) is based on ultrasonic imaging using a unique liquid film as a detector. The longitudinal ultrasonic waves are converted to an optical diffraction grating at the interface of the liquid film. The field of view of the system is about 8 x 10 cm with a resolution of about 1 and 1.7 mm at the operating frequencies of 5 and 3 MHz, respectively. The imaging is performed at the normal video rate of 30 frames per second. A complex flow of dense silica/water slurry up to the maximum packing solid fraction is readily imaged through a depth of 2.5 cm. The attenuation can be used for determining the concentration distribution within the flow field. Using spatial cross-correlation, the velocity of the moving textures in a heterogeneous flow field can be determined. This contribution will show details of the measurement approach and give results on concentration and velocity measurements.

[D.8]   Development of Mixing Models Using Resistance Tomography

R. Mann[1], R. A. Williams[2], T. Dyakowski[1], F. J. Dickin[3], and R. B. Edwards[4]

[1] *Department of Chemical Engineering, UMIST, P.O. Box 88, Manchester M60 1QD U.K.*

[2] *Camborne School of Mines, University of Exeter, Redruth, Cornwall TR15 3SE U.K.*

[3] *Department of Electrical Engineering and Electronics, UMIST, P.O. Box 88, Manchester M60 1QD U.K*

[4] *Unilever Research Port Sunlight Laboratory, Quarry Road East, Bebington, Wirral L63 3JW U.K.*

The application of Electrical Resistance Tomography (ERT) to visualize the mixing of solid-liquid, liquid-liquid, and gas-liquid systems at a laboratory and a pilot scale will be described. The wealth of data provided by ERT allows a fresh and radical approach to be taken in the development of mechanistic models that are capable of describing the distribution of the dispersed phase in three dimensions. This will be illustrated using a cellular flow model based on a network-of-zones. The utility of ERT to verify and develop the modeling procedures is demonstrated. Possible future applications of the technology and their implications for process engineering will be reviewed.

[D.9]   The Experimental Research of ECT Systems

B. F. Zhang, D. Y. Yao, and L. H. Peng

Department of Automation, Tsing-Hua University, Beijing 100084 China

This poster describes the test of a 10-electrode capacitance tomography system, including a static test using physical models and a dynamic test in a fluidized device. A method for evaluating the performance of the ECT system and the results of this evaluation are presented.

[D.10]   Nuclear Magnetic Resonance Imaging for Multiphase Flow Visualization

S. A. Altobelli, A. Capriban, E. Fukushima, D. O. Kuethe, and M. Nakagawa
The Lovelace Institutes, Albuquerque, New Mexico U.S.A.

Nuclear Magnetic Resonance Imaging (NMRI) is a popular technique in clinical medicine used to examine static objects. It is non-invasive, penetrates many optically opaque samples, has no preferred directions, and is relatively fast. We have used NMRI to study multiphase flows whereby advantage is taken of other virtues of the method, namely, its ability to measure many parameters and its ability to make measurements on flowing streams. The primary parameters measured are velocity and concentration of the separate phases. In addition it is possible to measure acceleration, diffusion, turbulence, and turbulence diffusivity. We have measured flows of pure liquids in pipes, foams, suspensions of particles in liquid, and two-phase immiscible liquids. We present some examples of such measurements and indicate the practical ranges for flow and imaging parameters. We will also discuss future capabilities such as high speed imaging by NMRI.

Session E: Separation and Reactor Technology

[E.1]   Multiphase Flow Characteristics of Air-Sparged Hydrocyclone Flotation as Revealed by X-Ray CT Analysis

J. D. Miller and A. Das

Department of Metallurgical Engineering, University of Utah, Salt Lake City,
     Utah 84112 U.S.A.

Air-sparged hydrocyclone technology is a new separation technology for the flotation separation of fine particles and involves the attendant complexities of three phase flow. In this regard, x-ray CT analysis has been used to describe multiphase flow characteristics and, based on radial density profiles, identify important flow regimes including the air core, froth phase, and swirl layer during quartz flotation.

[E.2]   A Study on LARCODEM Separators Using Electrical Resistance Tomography

M. Wang[1], F. J. Dickin[1], R. A. Williams[2], and T. Dyakowski[3]

[1] *Department of Electrical Engineering and Electronics, UMIST, P.O. Box 88, Manchester M60 1QD U.K.*

[2] *Camborne School of Mines, University of Exeter, Redruth, Cornwall TR15 3SE U.K.*

[3] *Department of Chemical Engineering, UMIST, P.O. Box 88, Manchester M60 1QD U.K.*

Centrifugal separation of solid and liquid is widely employed in chemical engineering. In the hydrocyclone the continuous fluid is water, whereas in dense medium separators (DMS) the continuous phase is a dense fluid such as a suspension of fine magnetite or ferrosilicon. The large coal dense medium separator (LARCODEMS) is a centrifugal dense medium separator developed for coal cleaning processes. Typically, a LARCODEMS 1.2 m in diameter and 3.6 m long could treat raw coal from 0.5 mm to 100 mm in diameter at a maximum feed rate of 250 tons per hour. An air core is present during operation of the separator, the importance of which has been recognized recently.

Electrical Impedance Tomography (EIT) provides a convenient means to measure and image the air core in hydrocyclone separators and in LARCODEMS on-line. The concentration of particles in a solid-liquid separation can also be imaged with the technique. However, present image reconstruction algorithms distort the size of the air core and the detailed concentration of the solids. A series of air core images presented in the paper are reconstructed with an iterative algorithm based on minimizing the error between the measured boundary voltages and the voltages predicted by the forward solution from an estimated core position. A means of estimating the diameter of the air core will be presented, which can be used for control of the separators.

The study demonstrates that EIT is capable of delivering on-line information on the geometry and the dynamics of air core movement and the relative changes in the solids concentration in centrifugal separation.

[E.3] Experience of Imaging and Tracking Positron-Emitting Tracers in Industrial Processes

D. J. Parker, D. M. Benton, T. D. Beynon, P. Fowles, and P. A. McNeil
School of Physics and Space Research, University of Birmingham,
Birmingham B15 2TT U.K.

The use of radioisotope tracers offers great flexibility for imaging, for example enabling the behavior of a single component of a multi-phase system to be observed. Radioisotopes that decay by positron emission have as their signature a pair of back-to-back γ-rays (originating from electron-positron annihilation), whose coincident detection can be used as the basis for tomographic reconstruction. At Birmingham a purpose-built "positron camera" has been used since 1985 for industrial imaging. Obtaining a full 3-D tomographic image of the distribution of a fluid tracer takes around an hour, but a single quantitative 2-D projected view can be measured in less than a minute. Alternatively, the new technique of Positron Emission Particle Tracking locates a single small tracer particle many times a second and is proving to be an extremely powerful tool for investigating flow and mixing within laboratory-scale equipment. This technique is currently being applied in studies of mixers and fluidized beds.

[E.4]   Gamma Densitometry Tomographic Measurements of Void Fraction and Spatial Distribution in Bubble Columns

K. A. Shollenberger, J. R. Torczynski, D. R. Adkins, and T. J. O'Hern

Engineering Sciences Center, Sandia National Laboratories, Albuquerque, New Mexico 87185-5800 U.S.A.

Hydrodynamic effects must be considered when attempting to scale slurry bubble-column reactors to sizes of industrial interest. However, the flows that occur in these opaque multiphase fluids are complex and not well characterized. The diagnostics typically used interfere with the flow, lack spatial resolution, or have yet to be applied under normal reactor operating conditions.

As part of the effort to assist in the design and scale-up of slurry-phase bubble-column reactors, non-invasive diagnostic techniques are being developed for measurements of gas hold-up. Gamma densitometry tomography (GDT) experiments have been performed on an air-water bubble column, a vertical Lucite® tube of 19 cm inner diameter with a non-rigid bubble-cap sparger. The GDT system uses a 5 Ci Cs-137 isotope source to provide a beam of 0.662 MeV gamma rays, which are detected using a sodium iodide (NaI) scintillation detector. The source and the detector are mounted on two opposing arms (with 60 cm clearance) of a heavy-duty, computer-controlled, two-axis transverse which has 60 cm of travel in both the horizontal and vertical directions. Operation of this system is fully automated.

Scans at a specific vertical position have been made for gas superficial velocities up to 12 cm/s, corresponding to average void fractions of up to 12%. The data was used to compute a axisymmetric "tomographic" reconstruction of the void fraction radial distribution. Void fractions was found to be greatest on the axis, decreasing monotonically to zero at the wall. Integration of these void-fraction profiles over the cross section was sued to obtain area-averaged void fraction results. To validate these results, the rise in the air-water interface during flow was measured so that the average void fraction for the whole column could be measured. These level-rise measurements agree reasonable well with the GDT results.

[E.5]   Two-Dimensional Imaging of Pulse Flow in Trickle-Bed Reactors Using Capacitance Tomography

N. Reinecke[1], C. G. Xie[2], D. Mewes[1], and M. S. Beck[3]

[1] *Institut für Verfahrenstechnik, Universität Hannover, Callinstraße 36*
        D-30167 Hannover, Germany

[2] *Schlumberger Cambridge Research, P.O. Box 153, Cambridge CB3 0HG U.K.*

[3] *Department of Electrical Engineering and Electronics, UMIST, P.O. Box 88,*
        Manchester M60 1QD U.K.

While some types of reactors found in the chemical industry use a single liquid phase, most of them are operated with a gaseous and a liquid phases flowing over a packing or catalyst. For certain flow rates of the two phases a pulse flow regime is established, which is attributed to the onset of instabilities of the liquid film covering the catalyst and the subsequent bridging of the voids between the packing. For small scale reactors these pulses cover the entire cross-sectional area of the reactor. Therefore the properties of the center of the pulse, especially in the front and back of the liquid slug, cannot be visually observed from the outside of the column.

In order to visualize the pulse flow in trickle-bed reactors, a 12-electrode sensor for capacitance tomography was used. The sensor is axially and radially guarded by grounded shields. The reconstruction on a 32 x 32 grid was conducted with a total of 66 linearly independent measurements gathered sequentially at a speed of 100 Hz. The capacitances were measured using a charge-transfer capacitance transducer, and the data acquisition was done by transputers installed in a host PC. The results show non-symmetrical properties of the liquid pulses. The properties of the pulses are largely dependent on the liquid distribution at the head of the column, even though an entrance length of about eight times the diameter of the column was maintained. An increase of the liquid film thickness at the back of the pulse as well as a decrease at the front of the pulse was observed. It was found that the initiation of a pulse often leads to a group of up to three pulses traversing the column together. A coalescence of pulses was not observed along the measurement length used in these experiments.

[E.6]   Visualization of Size-Dependent Segregation in Solid-Liquid Mixers Using Positron Emission Tomography

S. L. McKee[1], D. J. Parker[2], and R. A. Williams[3]

[1] *Department of Chemical Engineering, UMIST, P.O. Box 88, Manchester M60 1QD U.K.*

[2] *School of Physics and Space Research, University of Birmingham, Birmingham B15 2TT U.K.*

[3] *Camborne School of Mines, University of Exeter, Redruth, Cornwall TR15 3SE U.K.*

By labeling particles of specific sizes, it is possible to investigate the mixing behavior of solid-liquid slurries using positron emission tomography (PET). Solid concentration maps can be obtained under different mixing conditions (impeller speed, solids concentration, particle size distribution, *etc*). Experimental measurements for polydisperse and bimodal silica/water mixtures have been performed. The data obtained can be used to calculate the homogeneity of mixing and the segregation of particulates under different processing conditions. The results demonstrate the usefulness of PET to assist in the design of solid-liquid mixers. The method can be used on process-scale design and scale-up studies.

Session F: Characterization of Material Structure

[F.1]   Mass Transport Studied with Magnetic Resonance Imaging

L. D. Hall, T. A. Carpenter, G. Amin, J. A. Derbyshire, A. E. Fisher, K. Potter, D. Xing, A. R. C. Gates, B. Newling, R. G. Wise, and S. J. Gibbs
Herchel Smith Laboratory, Cambridge University School of Clinical Medicine, University Forvie Site, Robinson Way, Cambridge CB2 2PZ U.K.

Magnetic Resonance (MR) techniques offer a non-invasive means for obtaining images, in two or three dimensions, which are sensitive to molecular motions over a unique range of length and time scales in complex systems composed of water, hydrocarbons, or mixtures thereof. Of specific interest here are two MR windows for studying mass transport: serial MR imaging and pulsed field gradient spin-echo (PGSE) based techniques. Serial MR imaging permits observation of motions on a length scale of 0.01 to 10 cm and on a time scale of milliseconds to hours. It is thus useful for observing the evolution of unsteady systems, for example interdiffusion and chemical reaction. PGSE methods are sensitive to motions on a length scale of 0.1 to 100 microns and a time scale of milliseconds to seconds and can provide reliable measures of local velocities ranging from 100 μm/s to 1 m/s. Together these MR methods provide a powerful means of studying both molecular diffusion and flow, especially when coupled with a fast imaging protocol such as echo planar imaging (EPI).

This paper provides a summary of our recent uses of these MR techniques to monitor interdiffusion and to perform fluid velocimetry. Serial imaging has been used to map the temporal evolution of pH, redox potential, and paramagnetic ion concentration in hydrocolloid gels, paramagnetic ion migration in the brine-curing of meat, clay invasion of soil, and water infiltration into soil. Fluid velocimetry has been performed by PGSE methods in systems ranging in complexity from steady, one-dimensional, fully developed pipe flow to time-dependent, fully three-dimensional flows. Examples of the latter include pulsatile flow in elastic vessels, single phase flow in model porous media, and three-dimensional flows around baffles and manifolds.

[F.2] Use of Magnetic Resonance Imaging as a Viscometer for Process Monitoring

M. J. McCarthy, R. L. Powell, and K. McCarthy
Department of Food Science and Technology, University of California, Davis, California 95616 U.S.A.

The purpose of this paper is to introduce a rheometer that combines magnetic resonance imaging (MRI) flow measurements with fundamental principles of capillary flow. This technique can be used to obtain data over at least two decades of shear rates from a single point measurement. The measurement consists of a combined MRI velocity profile-pressure drop reading, producing over 128 data points over two or three decades of shear rate.

We view the primary application of this technique to be in monitoring on-line rheological properties of materials. This technique can be applied to opaque or transparent systems. Applications that will be presented include thermoplastics, tomato paste, and high density suspensions. Since the measurement is spatially resolved, multilayer studies can also be studied.

[F.3]   The Potential of MR Tomography in Assessing Mixing Quality

E. G. Smith[1], R. Kohli[2], P. A. Martin[2], J. W. Rockliffe[1], and T. Instone[1]

[1] *Unilever Research, Port Sunlight Laboratory, England, U.K.*

[2] *Magnetic Resonance Research Centre, University of Liverpool, England, U.K.*

The processing of many household products such as soap, creams, liquid detergents, and foods involves mixing and other dynamic events between a variety of physical states ranging from solutions and viscous liquids to liquid crystals and solid particles. By virtue of molecular mobility differences between these phases, NMR has found wide ranging application in studies of phase composition and thermal transitions in these materials. These studies have of necessity been confined to average measurements on bulk systems; however the recent transfer of Magnetic Resonance Imaging (MRI) technology from Medicine to Industry now makes it feasible to examine these processes spatially, in ways that are non-invasive and potentially quantitative.

While advances in fast MRI techniques (in particular Echo Planar Imaging) begin to satisfy the requirements for MR Tomography of dynamic processes, a comprehensive MRI technique to perform quantitative imaging of multi-phase mixing with capabilities of speed, high resolution, and solids detection is some way off. In the present work, using conventional MRI techniques and simple single phase viscous liquids, we explore the effects of the local variations in the physical state, concentration, or composition on contrast, and we evaluate how these effects can be used quantitatively in the study of mixing quality.

Standard spin echo MRI sequences on a GE 1.5 Tesla whole body scanner and a Bruker Micro Imager have been used to obtain T_2 and T_1 relaxation time weighted 2-D images of model liquids (glycerol and paramagnetically doped glycerol/water) undergoing laminar shear in two mixing geometries: rotating concentric cylinders and repetitive orifice flow. For laminar shear, MRI is able to visualize the mixing patterns and measure the striation thickness down to 200 microns. By suitable calibration measurements of T_1 and T_2 on known mixtures, MRI contrast has been converted into quantitative information about local concentration and domain integrity as a function of mixing cycles and diffusion time. In the case of orifice flow mixing, histograms of concentration population obtained by pixel sampling across the MR images provide a quantitative assessment of the dependence of mixing quality on orifice geometry. Preliminary results have been obtained for the diffusive mixing of water and liquid crystal-forming surfactant that demonstrate the potential of MRI mapping in studies of the spatial dynamics of phase formation under non-equilibrium and real-time conditions.

[F.4]   Microelectrical   Resistance   Imaging   of   Flowing Colloidal   Dispersions

R. A. Williams[1], P. J. Gregory[1], S. P. Luke[1], F. J. Dickin[2], L. Gate[3], and S. P. Taylor[4]

[1] Camborne School of Mines, University of Exeter, Redruth, Cornwall TR15 3SE U.K.

[2] Department of Electrical Engineering and Electronics, UMIST, P.O. Box 88, Manchester M60 1QD U.K.

[3] English China Clays International Research and Development, John Keay House, St. Austell, Cornwall PL25 4DJ U.K.

[4] BP Group Research and Engineering Centre, Chertsy Road, Sunbury-on-Thames, Middlesex TW16 7LN U.K.

Recent developments in the miniaturization of electrical resistance tomography will be described. By scaling down the technology that has been applied successfully to process pipes and vessels, it is possible to obtain information on the conductivity distribution within small tubes down to 1 mm in diameter. This technique involves the use of small sensing electrodes mounted on the inside periphery of the tube, a means of exciting those electrodes to obtain tomographic data, and reconstruction of the measured data taking into account wall conductance effects.

The technique, although at an early stage of development, would appear to have many potential applications in process and medical engineering. Two specific examples will be presented: monitoring of the state of dispersion of a liquid-liquid emulsion system, including measurement of the size and profile of coalesced droplets, and monitoring the state of aggregation and particle shape in clay dispersions.

[F.5]   X-Ray CT for On-Line Washability Analysis in Coal Preparation Plants

C. L. Lin[1], J. D. Miller[1], G. H. Luttrell[2], and G. T. Adel[2]

[1] *Department of Metallurgical Engineering, University of Utah, Salt Lake City, Utah 84112 U.S.A*

[2] *Department of Mining and Mineral Engineering, Virginia Polytechnic Institute and State University, Blacksburg, Virginia 24061 U.S.A.*

In view of the success of recent laboratory studies using x-ray CT to determine coal washability and with the availability of high speed CT systems, it now seems possible to design an on-line washability system for coal preparation plants. Design features for such a system are examined, and possible control strategies are discussed for different applications.

[F.6]   3-D Analysis and Simulation of Mineralogical Ores Using X-Ray and Neutron Micro-Tomography

R. A. Williams[1], E. J. Morton[2], X. Jia[1], and K. Atkinson[1]

[1] *Camborne School of Mines, University of Exeter, Redruth, Cornwall TR15 3SE U.K.*

[2] *Department of Physics, University of Surrey, Guildford, Surrey GU2 5XH U.K.*

The use of micro-tomographic techniques for 3-D tomographic analysis of whole ore specimens will be reviewed. These methods offera new a radically different approach to the quantitative analysis of minerals. The data obtained enable the likely comminution characteristics of the ores to be assessed <u>directly</u> without recourse to laborious microscopic analysis of 2-D polished sections and the consequent stereological uncertainty in using 2-D data (mineral phase sizes, phase contact perimeters, *etc.*) to reconstruct the true 3-D ore structure. The tomographic approach allows detailed 3-D computer simulations of ore structure to be developed and validated. The incentive for such simulations is that once visualizations of simple and complex ore structures are available, it is then possible to characterize completely the ore microstructure and consequent properties. For instance, the ore may be subjected to stress simulation analysis to predict its breakage and likely liberation characteristics.

Examples of preliminary microtomographic images and ore texture simulation results for a banded iron ore and a weathered granite will be presented.

[F.7]   NMR Rheometry

S. J. Gibbs[1], B. Newling[1], L. D. Hall[1], S. Ablett[2], W. Frith[2], and D. E. Haycock[2]

[1] *Herchel Smith Laboratory, Cambridge University School of Clinical Medicine,*
    University Forvie Site, Robinson Way, Cambridge CB2 2PZ U.K.

[2] *Unilever Research Laboratories, Colworth House, Sharnbrook,*
    Bedfordshire MK44 1LQ U.K.

Nuclear Magnetic Resonance (NMR) velocimetric imaging provides a unique opportunity for studying opaque fluid rheology under conditions of interest to process engineering. In this poster, NMR velocimetric methods are demonstrated for observing detailed velocity profiles in fully developed pipe flow. Systems examined include Newtonian liquids (water and aqueous sucrose solutions), polymer solutions, oil-in-water emulsions, and stable dispersions of small particles in oil and water. In addition to addressing a few technical issues concerning reliable NMR velocimetry, we consider two rheological problems: observing apparent wall slip and measuring shear-rate dependence of the fluid viscosity from the velocity profiles.

Apparent wall slip occurs when, because of steric and other effects, the dispersed phase is excluded from a thin layer of the fluid near the wall; as a result, this thin layer exhibits a markedly reduced viscosity compared with the bulk phase. Consequently, the thin *slip layer* exhibits very high shear, and the bulk velocity profile (extrapolated to the wall) shows a non-zero wall velocity. Detection of this apparent slip velocity by NMR imaging is discussed, and data are presented for the systems mentioned above.

For fully developed Poiseuille flow, the viscosity is proportional to the ratio of the radial coordinate to the radial derivative of the fluid velocity, where the constant of proportionality is one half the pressure drop per unit length of tubing. By differentiating NMR measured velocity profiles in the radial direction and measuring the pressure drop in the pipe due to flow, the shear-rate dependence of the fluid viscosity may be determined. Results are presented for the systems list above and compared with results from conventional cone-and-plate rheometry.

Author Index

Subject Index